An Illustrated Guide to Personal Health

An Illustrated Guide to Personal Health

How to Improve Your Health in Forty Common-Sense Steps

Tom Emerick & Robert Woods
Illustrated by Madi Schmidt

ISBN: 1511978236
ISBN 13: 9781511978231
Library of Congress Control Number: 2015907027
CreateSpace Independent Publishing Platform
North Charleston, South Carolina

CONTENTS

INTRODUCTION

Few things are more important to each of us than our personal health. If you don't have good health, not much else matters.

Most Americans look to their doctors to keep them healthy. In short, most of us are "medicalizing" our lives. That is a big mistake. Period. You may like your doctor. You may love your doctor. But half of all doctors are below average. (Unless they live in Lake Wobegon, of course.)

Doctors are pretty good about treating you when you're sick. But they really can't do much to give you greater well-being or make you healthier.

Alas, medical care can really only deal with about 20 to 25 percent of the things that can cause you to die before your time.

The remaining 75 to 80 percent of health risks come from such factors as genetics, lifestyle, contentment, resilience, a satisfying job, social connections, and good relationships with friends and family. Aside from genetics, you alone can control 75 to 80 percent of the things that may cause you to die early.

Serious job dissatisfaction is a killer. If you have a job you hate, you have three choices: (1) try to learn to like your job; (2) quit and find a job you can tolerate, or even enjoy, even if the pay is less; or (3) be prepared to suffer a lot of illness and probably die early. No doctor can treat job misery.

Life is a journey during which we all face an abundance of stresses. One important key to good health is learning to cope well with stress. Be resilient. Learn how to bounce back. Try to keep a good sense of humor through life's ups and downs. You will be healthier and enjoy the journey more, as well.

Harboring anger is a killer. It's corrosive to your soul. Forgive early and forgive often. Living with anger and resentment harms you in many ways.

As this book will show, being lonely is a huge health risk. Your doctor does not have a pill for loneliness and never will. You and you alone are in control of this. In every community, there are places you are always welcome. You've just got to get off your sofa and find them. The rewards are huge.

If you get the best medical care possible, and the other 75 to 80 percent of risk factors are out of control, you'll probably lead an unhealthy life. You will not be well or have any sense of well-being.

This book is about how to address the health risks you can control. We will show you forty things you can start doing today to get control of your health and well-being.

By the way, gaining control of your life risks—rather than depending on doctors to control them for you—will probably make you feel liberated and less stressed-out.

This book will show you that you have an abundance of options and choices to have a healthier, happier life.

The cost of health care in the United States is simply unsustainable. Medicare and Medicaid are woefully underfunded for the next twenty years. The costs of private health-insurance plans continue to go up and up. However, if everyone did what he or she could to be healthier, we could extend the funding of our health care.

The authors of this book have a favor to ask. If you happen to meet our personal doctors—a long shot, we know—please don't tell them about this book. The last thing anyone needs is a hacked-off doctor doing a colorectal exam on you.

Warning: As you read this book, you will see a lot of repetitive redundancy, over and over. Why? We are trying to inculcate you with certain principles. ("Inculcate" is an old-fashioned word meaning to teach by pounding something into people's heads.) If you're reading this book, it's too late. You've already paid for it.

Another warning: Much of what we have written here is documented science. The problem is so-called scientific studies in health care are often contradictory. For example, a certain vitamin supplement may raise your risk of cancer according to one study, but another study says the same vitamin may lower your risk of heart disease. What do you do? Since we all have a hundred or more health risk factors--the combinations and permutations of which are mind-boggling--we just have to do the best we can.

Some of what we wrote here is less science than a merger of philosophy and personal observations. None of us can know the hour of our passing, but we can do our best to enjoy the time we have and to do the best by others. This notion is reflected throughout this book.

Sometimes our cited statistics don't match up. One study reports 70 percent of something, and another study of the same thing reports 72 percent. We are aware of this but decided to report each study's results faithfully. We didn't fiddle with the numbers to make them consistent.

Some people do almost everything wrong their entire lives, and we mean *everything*, and live to be age ninety.

ACKNOWLEDGMENTS

Even though this is only a small book, it would not have been a book at all without the help of some other people.

In this book, we emphasize how friendships can be important to your happiness and health. The authors of *An Illustrated Guide to Managing Your Health* have been dear friends for over fifty years. We, Tom and Bob, would like to acknowledge each other for a lifetime of friendship and priceless conversations and inspiration.

Fortunately, we have had many lifelong friends from whom we've learned much about resilience, hard work, integrity, loyalty, and good humor.

Special thanks go to Madi Schmidt, who created the illustrations for this book.

We are indebted to Tom's wife, Patricia, and Bob's wife, Laura, who were invaluable in editing and telling us when we were way off base. We cannot thank them enough.

The books written by Nortin Hadler, MD, have been a great source of both philosophy and science. His books have been most influential to us.

The folks at CreateSpace, our publisher, have been absolutely terrific. They're fast and efficient.

All errors and omissions are entirely our own.

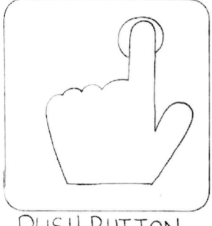

PUSH BUTTON

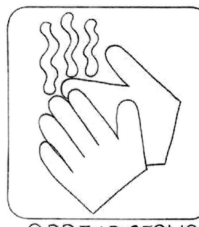

SPREAD GERMS

CHAPTER 1

AVOID HAND DRYERS IN PUBLIC RESTROOMS

Anyone's life truly lived consists of work, sunshine, exercise,
soap, plenty of fresh air, and a happy contented spirit.
—LILLIE LANGTRY

In public restrooms, the way you dry your hands is important. Have you used those electric hand dryers common in public restrooms today—you know, the ones that say how hygienic they are? Well, have you ever considered the source of the air that is blowing your hands dry? Is it piped in from Hawaii or Tahiti or from an oxygen tank somewhere? Of course not: It is air from inside the bathroom. So, in effect, you are drying your clean hands with bathroom air.

Floating around public restrooms are all manner of bacteria and viruses. Some are really nasty stuff. The hand dryers basically inhale a huge volume of germ-laden air and blow it all over your wet hands so the germs can dry and stick to your hands. Yuck. Yuck. Yuck.

In 2013, researchers unleashed a harmless germ not ordinarily found in restrooms and then tested for its presence in various parts of the restroom. The counts of that germ were twenty-seven times higher near the hand dryers.[1]

In addition, a study published in the *Journal of Applied Microbiology* in 2011 showed that paper towels consistently outperformed hand dryers.[2]

Here's another public-potty tip. Many people do not wash their hands after they use the john. Try not to touch the inside handle of a public-restroom door with your bare hands. Use a paper towel or the edge of your jacket or shirt.

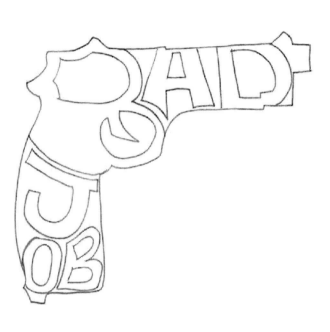

CHAPTER 2

JOB MISERY IS A KILLER

Oh, you hate your job? Why didn't you say so? There's a support group for that. It's called everybody, and they meet at the bar.
—George Carlin

If you hate your job, either learn to tolerate it or find a new job. Seventy percent of Americans reported disliking their jobs.[3] Hating your job has negative consequences, including weight gain, weakened immune systems, ruined relationships (with coworkers and family), loss of sleep, risk of serious injury, and increased aging.[4]

Hating is also transferable. It rubs off on others. Before you act like you hate your job and display frequent anger as a result, think about the effect this will have on your family and children, now and in their futures. Children mimic their parents. Acting this way may make your kids unhappy haters too.[5]

No job is 100 percent positive all the time. As Dan Pink says in his TED Talk, real motivation does not come from traditional rewards.[6] Motivation comes from accomplishing something you truly desire. Move on if you are not in a job you either enjoy or can tolerate.

Two people can have identical jobs; one may hate it while the other really likes it. Mike Rowe, the star of *Dirty Jobs*, once said, "Don't wait for your job to give you passion, take your passion to your job."

Steve Jobs, the founder of Apple, noted, "Your work is going to fill a large part of your life, and the only way to be truly satisfied is to do what you believe is great work. And the only way to do great work is to love what you do. If you haven't found it yet, keep looking. Don't settle. As with all matters of the heart, you'll know when you find it. And, like any great relationship, it just gets better and better as the years roll on."

By the way, any job done for an honest living deserves respect.

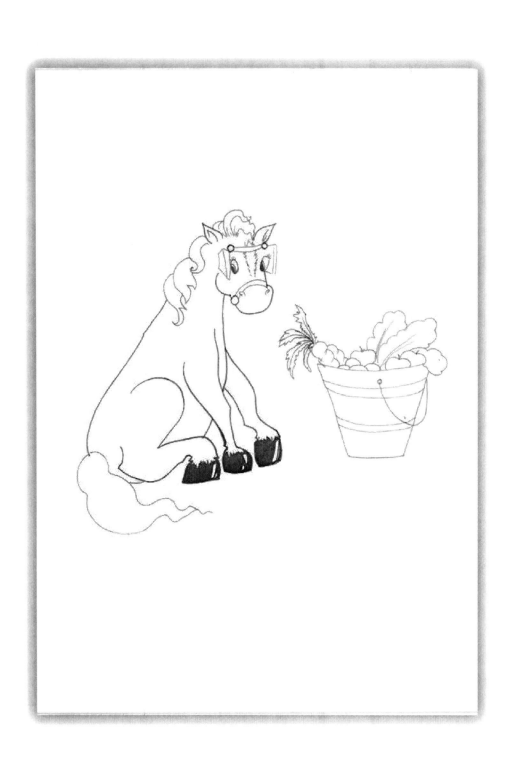

CHAPTER 3

IGNORE FAD DIETS

*The second day of a diet is always easier than
the first. By the second day you're off it.*
—Jackie Gleason

A fad diet is any program that promises quick weight loss through an unusual approach to eating. Most promise weight loss without exercise.

The University of Pittsburgh Medical Center asks patients to answer these questions before starting a diet:

- Does the diet promise quick weight loss?
- Does the diet sound too good to be true?
- Does the diet help sell a company's product?
- Does the diet lack valid scientific research to support its claims?
- Does the diet give lists of "good" and "bad" foods?

If the answer to *any* of these questions is yes, then it is a fad diet.[7]

Fad diets are targeted at people who want to lose weight quickly without exercise. But the losses are usually short-term and/or due to losing water weight. The basic fact is we eat too much food. Two-thirds of US adults and one-third of children are overweight or obese. Fad diets cannot cure that, and in fact, many are dangerous to your health. Many fad diets can cause dangerous spikes in blood sugar as well as increases in cholesterol and blood-pressure levels.[8]

Take the advice of the Centers for Disease Control (CDC). The CDC says the key to achieving and maintaining a healthy lifestyle isn't about making short-term dietary changes. Instead, adopt a lifestyle that includes healthful eating and regular physical activity. Nothing else really works.

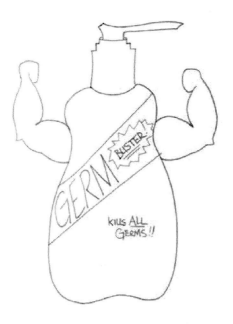

CHAPTER 4

AVOID ANTIBACTERIAL SOAPS AND GELS

Soap and water and common sense are the best disinfectants.
—WILLIAM OSLER

Overuse of antibacterial soaps and gels can reduce the effectiveness of antibiotics you may need someday. They are helping create antibiotic-resistant germs.

Triclosan and triclocarban are two chemicals included in antibacterial soaps, and both are endocrine disruptors—meaning they pose a risk of disrupting the thyroid, which can potentially disrupt metabolism and cause weight gain. A study published in *Environmental Science and Technology* found triclosan in 100 percent of the women's urine samples and triclocarban in 87 percent of all samples. That's a definite health risk.[9]

It is hard to get away from antibacterial products. Most soaps today contain an antibacterial ingredient. Allison Aiello, PhD, an epidemiology professor at the University of Michigan, studied people who washed their hands with regular or antibacterial soap and found "there was no difference between groups, either in bacteria on the hands or in rates of illness."[10]

So find some regular soap and use it instead of the antibacterial type. You may even save money.

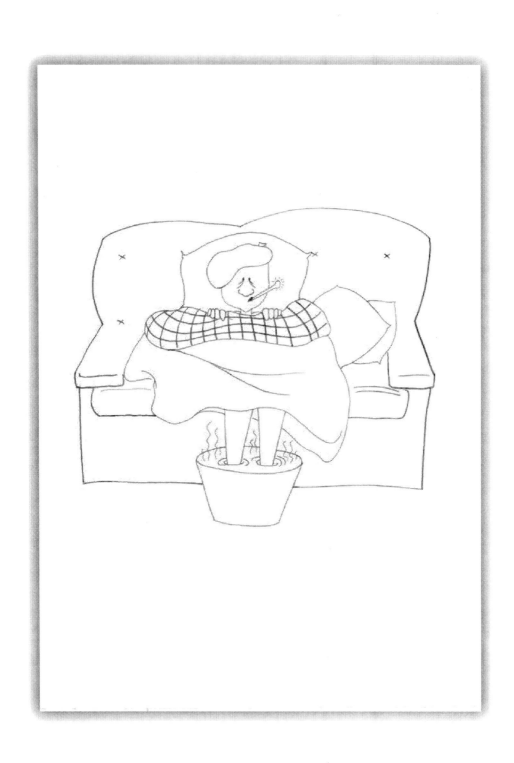

CHAPTER 5

DON'T GO TO THE DOCTOR FOR A COLD

If you take antibiotics for a cold you will get better in a week. If you don't, you will get better in seven days.
—ANONYMOUS

Going to see a doctor for a cold is a waste of time and money. On average, adults get two to five colds per year. Children get as many as seven to ten. That means Americans get about one billion colds per year. Going to a doctor every time you have one does not help. Your body will likely recover on its own.

As is commonly believed, you should go to the doctor if you have a prolonged, high fever (102°F for adults, 103°F for children), symptoms that last more than ten days, trouble breathing, pain or pressure in the chest, confusion or disorientation, severe or persistent vomiting, severe pain in the face or forehead, or if you faint or feel like you are about to faint. Also, go to the doctor if your child has either a bad earache or drainage from the ear.[11]

You can help reduce the number of colds you get by eating a healthy diet, exercising, and practicing basic sanitation (washing hands with soap, wiping counters, and not sharing glasses or other utensils). In addition, when you are ill, carefully clean every surface you touch so you won't spread your cold.

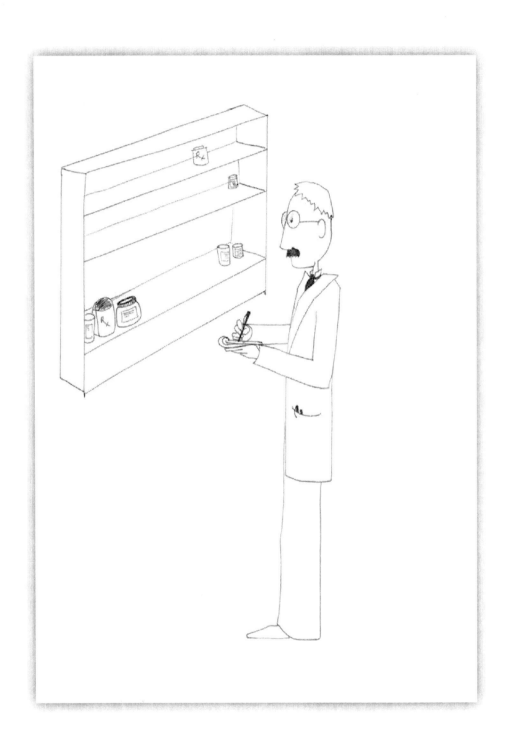

CHAPTER 6

ASK YOUR DOCTOR FOR GENERIC DRUGS

There is no medicine like hope, no incentive so great, and no
tonic so powerful as expectation of something tomorrow.
—ORISON SWETT MARDEN

You can save big using generic drugs. The average price of a generic drug is about fifteen dollars, while brand name drugs average eighty to one hundred dollars. Therefore, consumers save about 85 percent with generic drugs.

A generic drug is made with the same active ingredients and is available in the same strength and dosage as the equivalent brand-name drug. In fact, a generic drug is identical—or bioequivalent—to a brand-name drug in dosage form, safety, strength, administration, quality, performance characteristics, and intended use. Generic drugs save consumers an estimated $8 to $10 billion a year at retail pharmacies. Even more billions are saved when hospitals use generics.[12]

A recent study showed that doctors often prescribe brand-name drugs simply because patients ask for them. Of course, these are the drugs the patients see on television, and they don't know the generic names for the same drugs.[13]

Walmart offers a growing list of generic drugs at a price of four dollars per script. That may be well below your out-of-pocket copay for a branded drug. Pharmacy chains such as Walgreens are offering low-priced generic drugs too. Over-the-counter drugs can also save you big money.

Don't listen to modern snake-oil salesmen who promote products as miracle cures. Many of these products are not tested and either have no effect or may cause more harm than good.[14]

Congress is finally beginning to crack down on products that don't help. If you want to know more about this, look up how Congress "burned" Dr. Mehmet Oz, one of the best-known physicians in the United States, who had been promoting one "miracle cure" after another.[15]

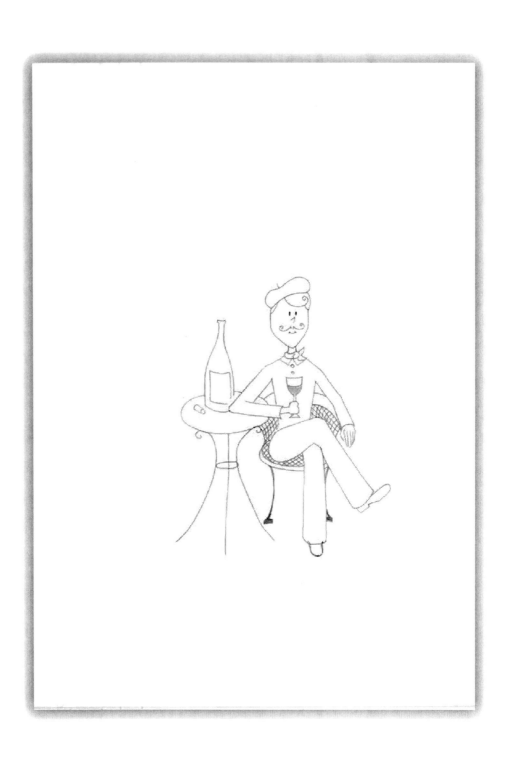

CHAPTER 7

DRINK A GLASS OF RED WINE DAILY

My wife and I really enjoy a glass of red wine. We're
too old to drink cheap wine, and we don't.
—Paul Henderson

R ed wine used in moderation is good for your health. It increases antioxidants.

Red wines help raise HDL—the "good" cholesterol. They also contain resveratrol, which helps prevent damage to blood vessels, reduces low-density lipoprotein (LDL) cholesterol (the "bad" cho-lesterol), and prevents blood clots.[16]

In fact, according to *The Journal of Physiology*, drinking a glass of wine is equivalent to an hour of exercise.[17]

Other alcohols may be equally preventative. Two researchers conducted a study in Northern California that followed 128,934 adults from 1978 to 1990 and found that people who had one or two alcoholic drinks per day have a 32 percent lower risk of dying of coronary heart disease than nondrinkers.[18]

If you're going to drink a glass of wine anyway, you may as well buy good wine and enjoy it. Enjoying life is good for you.

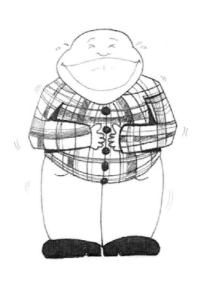

CHAPTER 8

LAUGHTER HEALS, BOREDOM KILLS

Laughter is an instant vacation.
—Milton Berle

L aughing is good for you in many ways. It's a great medicine that reduces anxiety and combats fear. It comforts you. It relaxes you. It reduces pain. It boosts the immune system. It reduces stress, creates optimism, and enhances communication.[19]

Laughter also relaxes your muscles, lowers your respiration rate, reduces your blood pressure, and is what Dr. Fry, MD and professor of psychiatry at Stanford University, refers to as "internal jogging," because one minute of laughter is equal to ten minutes on a rowing machine in terms of providing good cardiac, abdominal, facial, and back muscle conditioning.[20]

More than seven thousand civil servants in England were interviewed regularly over twenty-five years—and those who said they were bored were nearly 40 percent more likely to have died by the end of the study than those who did not.[21]

The researchers in the study believe the boredom-death connection might exist because bored people were more likely to feel unfulfilled, unmotivated, and unhappy, which could lead to unhealthful behaviors such as excessive drinking, smoking, overeating, and drug use. The state of boredom, they wrote, "is almost certainly a proxy for other risk factors."

Is this how you want to go out? Don't let boredom kill you.

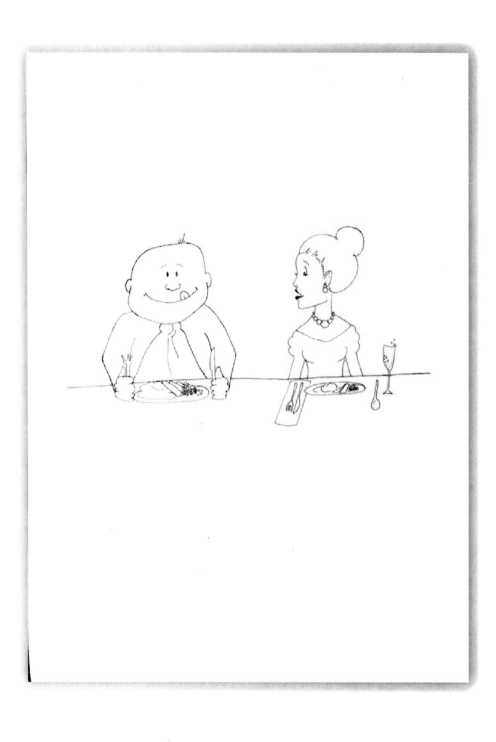

CHAPTER 9

GIVE YOUR FORK A REST

All you need is love. But a little chocolate
now and then doesn't hurt.
—CHARLES M. SCHULZ

Eating makes you feel good by releasing dopamine. Dopamine produces a sense of pleasure. But eating fast does not give your body time to make this transition.[22]

It takes about twenty minutes for your body to tell your brain it is full. A WebMD study of seventeen hundred women in Japan showed that eating slowly resulted in lower calorie consumption. Therefore, eating slowly helps you lose weight. People who ate lunch in ten minutes consumed an estimated 646 calories. Those who took twenty-five or more consumed only 579. This shows that more pleasure means fewer calories.

The Slow Food movement was formed twenty years ago in Italy to counter the fast-food industry. This group reports that eating slowly has several positive effects—including weight loss, better digestion, reduced stress, and, of course, more pleasure from enjoying your meal.[23]

Precision Nutrition reports that slow eaters consume about 2 ounces of food per minute, while fast eaters consume about 3.1 ounces per minute. Fast eaters also took larger bites and chewed less before swallowing.[24]

Eating fast can lead to choking. In the United States, twenty-five hundred people choke to death on food each year. The rate of choking goes up as people age. Eating fast while dining alone is also a risk simply because there is no one there to perform the Heimlich maneuver on you.

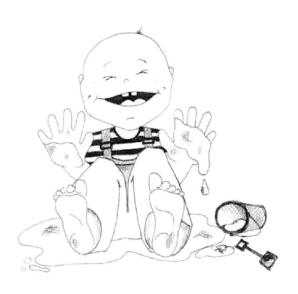

CHAPTER 10

LET KIDS PLAY IN DIRT

> *Dirt is good. If your child isn't coming in dirty every*
> *day, they are not doing their job. Playing in dirt*
> *builds an immunological army for the future.*
> —CBS NEWS, 2009

The CBS quote above refers to the "hygiene hypothesis." The hygiene hypothesis says that early exposure to parasites, bacteria, and viruses that you might get from playing in dirt helps prevent people from having allergies, asthma, and other autoimmune disorders during adulthood.

In fact, hygiene studies seem to explain why immune-system disorders such as multiple sclerosis, type 1 diabetes, inflammatory bowel disease, asthma, and allergies have risen significantly in the United States and other developed countries in recent years.[25]

Science magazine published an article about the same topic. *Science* noted that the rise in autoimmune diseases can be attributed to not allowing kids to develop strong immune systems when they are young.[26]

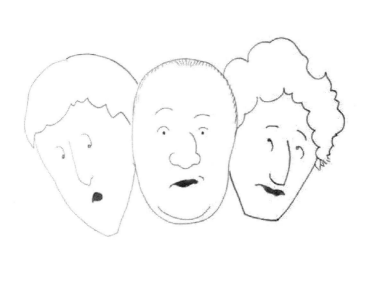

CHAPTER 11

ONE ACT OF STUPIDITY CAN WRECK YOUR LIFE

> *Never attribute to malice that which can be*
> *adequately explained by stupidity.*
> —ANONYMOUS

Seeing the Three Stooges or other comedians do stupid things is funny. Doing stupid things in real life is not only *not* funny but is also potentially career-disabling, marriage-wrecking, or dangerous to your health.

The list of people who have ruined their lives by doing one stupid thing is long. General Davis Petraeus had a brief affair with an aide and lied about it. This ruined his career as director of the CIA. Senator Gary Hart ruined his presidential bid by being caught on a boat named *Monkey Business* with his girlfriend.

Thomas Edison electrocuted a bunch of animals trying to win an argument with Nikola Tesla by proving that AC current was more dangerous than DC current. Animal-rights people never forgave him.

Why do people do stupid things? One study published in the *Journal of Personality and Social Psychology* noted people have what is called a "bias blind spot."

According to research, this bias blind spot is more likely to trip up smart people than average people. This is because smarter people are more likely to take shortcuts or make assumptions based on overconfidence.[27]

Again, an act of stupidity can wreck your health and your life.

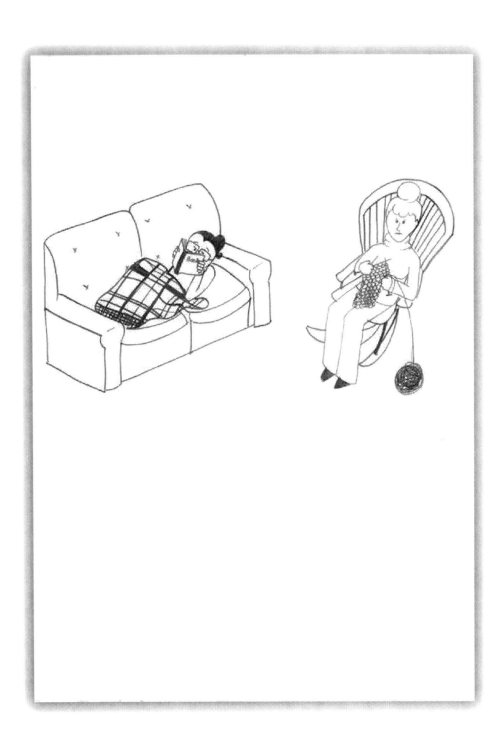

CHAPTER 12

ENJOY HOBBIES

I don't care to belong to any club that will have me as a member.
—GROUCHO MARX

Hobbies help everyone. Many people in their forties and fifties are so wrapped up in their work lives that they get very little mental relaxation or variation.

Hobbies are good for your health. Research has shown that hobbies reduce both stress and your waistline; they lower blood pressure and help you stay in the present.[28]

Hobbies can also unite you with others, and that helps provide the mental and physical conditioning necessary for a healthy life. If a hobby gets you away from the television—hurrah!

An online publication suggests ten popular hobbies to try. These are travel, volunteering, arts and crafts, music/theater/dance, clubs/associations, exercise, cooking, getting outside, teaching, and reconnecting with family. Others have suggested genealogy and family-history research.[29]

You may find that learning moderate exercises, helping to care for grandchildren, fostering an animal, serving as a crossing guard, or completing crossword or jigsaw puzzles help keep you busy. Each of these activities keeps your mind active and helps lower the risk of Alzheimer's disease.

Some people may enjoy creative hobbies such as painting, making birdhouses, sculpting, and writing. Others prefer more physical hobbies, such as gardening, swimming, running, hiking, golf, tennis, soccer, lacrosse, walking, and skiing. Each of these activities provides the benefits of stress reduction and exercise.

CHAPTER 13

SET GOALS

*If I had known that I would live this long, I
would have taken better care of myself.*
—EUBIE BLAKE, COMPOSER AND JAZZ PIANIST

In *Alice's Adventures in Wonderland*, the Cheshire Cat asked Alice where she wanted to go. Alice replied she did not know. To this the cat said, "Then any road will get you there."

Setting goals is important to making your life happier and more productive, both of which can help make you healthier.

Goals can be immediate, such as deciding what you want to get done today, or long-term, such as things to do when you retire. Productive people plan their day. People who get ahead nearly always set goals for themselves.

Complex goals are hard to attain. Consider the goal of losing a hundred pounds. That is a hard goal to achieve. It is a complex goal. To lose a hundred pounds, you have to do many things, including eating less, exercising more, and eating healthier.

Simple, more attainable goals would be better. For instance, a goal of eating more vegetables would help to attain the objective of losing a hundred pounds. So would a simple goal to exercise at least thirty minutes per day or to eat sweets only once or twice per week. These goals are more easily attainable and are therefore motivating.

If you have difficulty attaining goals, start small.

Goal attainment makes you feel good, builds self-esteem, and leads to good health.

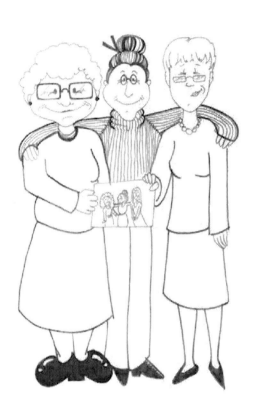

CHAPTER 14

HAVING FRIENDS MAY SAVE YOUR LIFE

A person doesn't measure his wealth by dollars and cents,
he measures his wealth by the number of friends he has.
—KELSEY PAIGE BOYD

Having many friends helps you be healthier. Surprisingly, friends are more important to your health than your family. This appears to be true at every age.

A study in Australia conducted by the Centre for Aging Studies looked at fifteen hundred elderly people for ten years. Those who had a large network of friends significantly outlived those with the fewest friends.[30]

Looking at the other end of the age spectrum, another study found that college freshmen who had small social networks and claimed to be lonely had weaker immune systems and higher levels of stress.[31]

The journal *Cancer* studied women with ovarian cancer and learned that those who had more friends and a better social network also had lower levels of a protein linked to a more aggressive form of breast cancer. Those women with high social support also were 70 percent less likely to develop this form of cancer.

A Stanford University study found that women who participated in support groups for social interaction lived twice as long as those who did not. A separate study on women with breast cancer found that socially isolated women had a 66 percent higher risk of death from all causes than those with social networks—and their breast-cancer death rate was twice as high.[32]

Studies have also shown that people with many friends live longer after heart attacks than people with few friends. Friends may even reduce your chances of getting a cold. However, be careful which friends you choose. A large 2007 study showed a nearly 60 percent increase in the risk of obesity among people whose friends gained weight.[33] One study showed that having many friendships helped reduce the risk of heart attack and fatal coronary heart disease. Relatives alone did not have the same effect.[34]

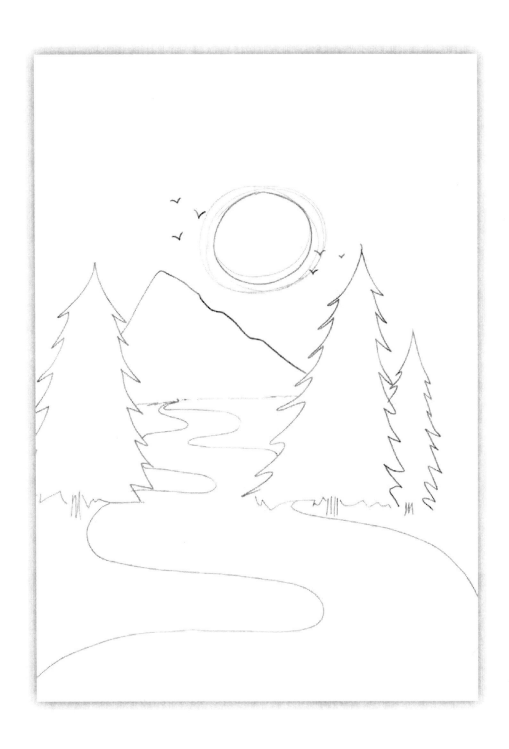

CHAPTER 15

ENJOY THE MOMENTS IN YOUR LIFE

*Life is not measured by the number of breaths we take but
rather by the moments that take your breath away.*
—ANONYMOUS

Staying "in the moment" helps improve your health. The experience of daily positive affect, or staying in the moment, even helps
patients with chronic diseases, including coronary artery disease,
high blood pressure, and asthma.

There's a 50 percent chance your mind is on something else as
you read this sentence. People daydream a lot. A Harvard study in
2010 asked people to track their thoughts, feelings, and activities at
random intervals and discovered they spent nearly half their time
doing one thing while thinking about another. They also found that
daydreaming makes them less happy than paying attention to the
present moment, even when it's unpleasant.[35]

Staying in the moment can be difficult. There are so many dis-
tractions. However, you can teach yourself to do so.

Learn to enjoy some moments every day. Enjoying a beautiful
sky, sunset, sunrise, or starry night is a stress reliever and helps make
life worthwhile. Savor that first cup of coffee in the morning slowly
and thoughtfully. If nothing else comes to mind, think about the
beautiful place where those coffee beans were grown.

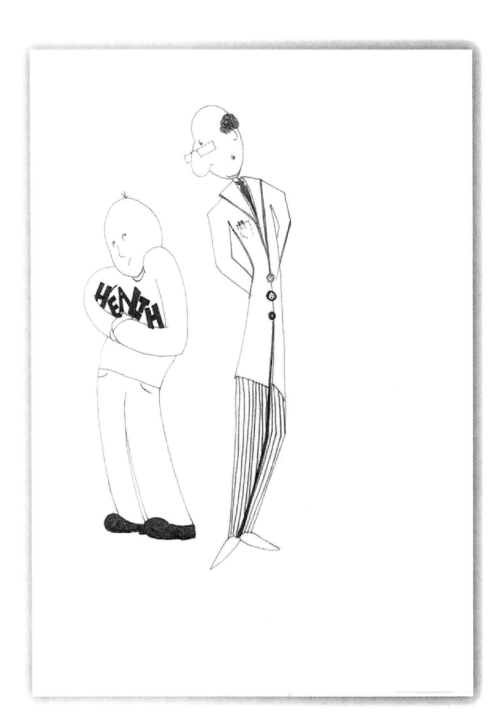

CHAPTER 16

DON'T TRUST YOUR HEALTH TO DOCTORS

An apple a day keeps the doctor away.
—Anonymous

The apple-a-day saying came from an era in which people wanted to avoid going to doctors. Today, many people think they should go to doctors early and often.

Doctors are who you want to see if you're sick. Doctors treat illnesses. However, they really can't do much to keep you healthy. Only you can control your health risks.

Half of all doctors in every country are below average. Americans have a tendency to trust their own doctors but mistrust the medical system as a whole. The United States ranked twenty-fourth in the world in terms of public trust in the overall health-care system. There is good reason to be skeptical. Each year, about four hundred thousand preventable drug-related injuries occur in US hospitals, according to the Institute of Medicine.[36]

Citizens of twenty-nine countries were asked two questions. The first asked about satisfaction with their last doctor visit. The United States ranked third on that question. Most Americans were satisfied with their last doctor visit.

The second asked about trust. When asked whether doctors in the United States could be trusted overall, a much lower opinion of doctors was reported. Here, the United States ranked twenty-fourth, tied with Croatia and behind Slovenia, Portugal, the Philippines, South Korea, and Slovakia, among others.[37]

An article in the prestigious *New England Journal of Medicine* reported Americans' opinions of the health-care system another way. According to the article, public trust in US doctors and medical leaders has declined sharply over the past half century, from 73 percent in 1966 to 34 percent in 2012.[38] For the record, Switzerland, Denmark, the Netherlands, and Britain ranked highest overall.

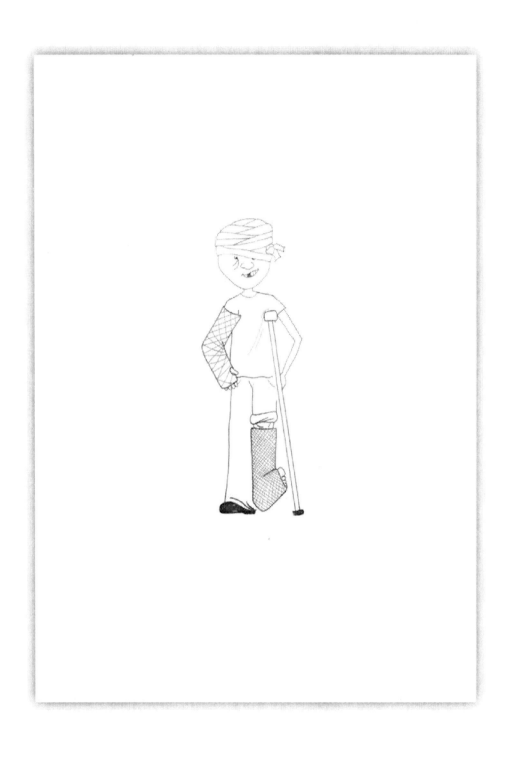

CHAPTER 17

AVOID SURGERY UNLESS YOU HAVE NO OTHER CHOICE

I've had so much plastic surgery, when I die
they will donate my body to Tupperware.
—JOAN RIVERS

All surgery is risky. The fact is too much surgery is done in America. According to a Mayo Clinic report, about 34 percent of elective surgery is unnecessary.[39]

Having unneeded surgery is a huge risk. If a doctor suggests surgery for you, you should first get a second opinion and then carefully consider whether you really need surgery. About a third of the time, the first doctor is wrong.

The *Journal of Patient Safety* noted that between 210,000 and 400,000 Americans die each year from "preventable medical harm." That makes bad medical care the third-highest cause of death in the United States. Many of these deaths involve unnecessary surgeries. Be especially wary of prescriptions for spine surgery, stents, cardiac bypass surgery, and arthroscopic knee surgery.[40]

In 2013, *USA Today* reported a story of a young professional baseball player who was told he needed a pacemaker. Later, the player found out the pacemaker was unnecessary, and doctors have since turned it off. In the meantime, however, the doctor performed many additional unnecessary surgeries and bilked Medicare out of millions of dollars. Fortunately, this doctor was caught and is now in prison.

Finally, if you must have surgery, you should know there are huge discrepancies among hospitals in terms of rates of infection and avoidable deaths. It's a good idea to check the hospital's Leapfrog safety scores. They are available online.[41]

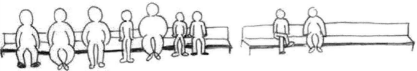
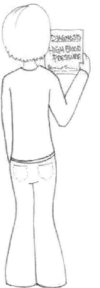

CHAPTER 18

BEWARE OF MISDIAGNOSES

*The biggest quality failure in health care
is to misdiagnose the patient.*
—ANONYMOUS

If you have a complex health problem, you stand a good chance of being misdiagnosed. This often happens when patients see multiple specialists who do not coordinate their treatments and diagnoses. Most people know a family member this has happened to.

If you are misdiagnosed, the treatment you get will be wrong. You won't get better and may have unnecessary surgery. Plus, you'll be subjected to unnecessary tests that are uncomfortable, painful, inconvenient, expensive, and intrusive.

"Overdiagnosis" is when you have a relatively minor health problem the doctor inflates to a more serious diagnosis. Overdiagnosis is dangerous to your health. Remember: half of all doctors in the United States are below average. Your doctor may be in the bottom 10 percent.

Examples of overdiagnoses are sometimes caused by changes in medical guidelines. For instance, after the criteria used to define osteoporosis were altered, seven million American women were turned into patients with a medical condition—literally overnight. The proliferation of fetal monitoring in the 1970s was associated with a 66 percent increase in the number of women told they needed emergency C-sections, though in fact many did not.

The introduction of prostate-cancer screening resulted in over a million additional American men being told they have prostate cancer, although in actuality many receive false positive reports from this test. A good book on prostate care is *Invasion of the Prostate Snatchers* by Mark Scholz and Ralph Blum.

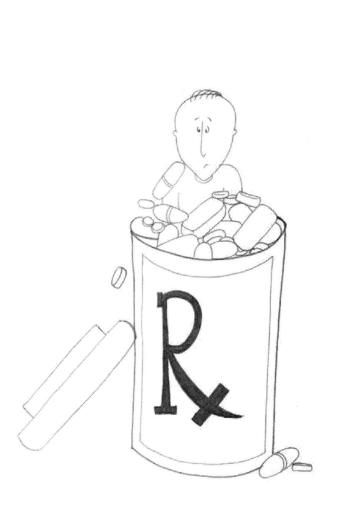

CHAPTER 19

AVOID OVERMEDICATION

Medicine acts as both remedy and poison.
—SOCRATES

Being overmedicated is common, and it is bad for your health. Many Americans are seriously overmedicated.

Nearly 30 percent of seniors take at least five medications a day. Many of these drugs may be good, but in some cases, we don't know the long-term effects. Consider Vioxx, the arthritis drug taken off the market after causing between 88,000 and 139,000 heart attacks in the five years it was sold.[42]

There are at least 1.5 million adverse drug events in the United States every year, thousands of them fatal.[43] One-third of these are among senior citizens. One problem is having multiple physicians taking care of various problems for a patient. Eighty-one percent of people with serious chronic conditions have two or more physicians, more than half have three or more, and a third have four or more, each one providing medications.[44]

NBC News reported a case of a sixty-one-year-old woman who was losing her memory. A specialist engaged to investigate identified twenty-seven different drug interactions among the woman's medications, most of moderate or high severity. In addition, a third of these could cause memory loss, confusion, or impaired cognition. Once off several of these medications, her memory problems ceased.[45] This cured her medically induced dementia.

Children are also overmedicated. About 1.3 percent of children are prescribed antidepressants, a six fold increase over the last twenty years.[46] The CDC estimates that 11 percent of children age four to seventeen have received a diagnosis of ADHD. According to Dr. Nancy Rappaport, a child psychiatrist in Boston, doctors are assuming kids have ADHD when sometimes the cause is just a rotten home environment.[47]

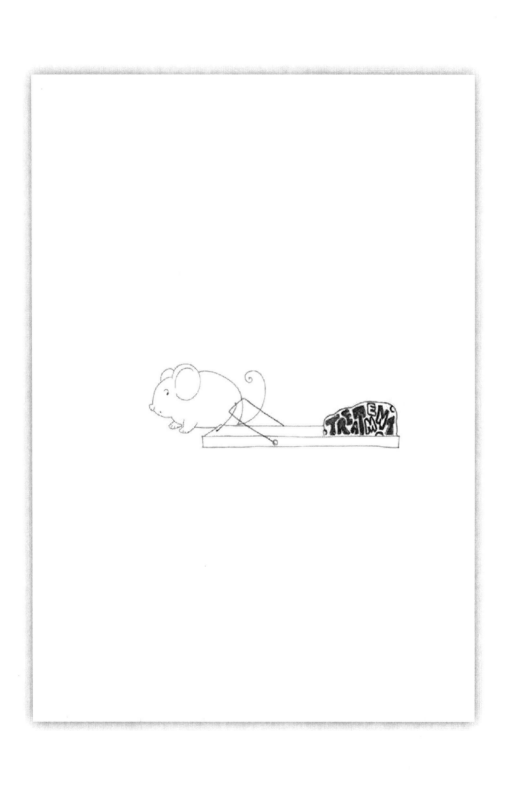

CHAPTER 20

AVOID TREATMENT TRAPS

When a lot of remedies are suggested for a
disease, that means it cannot be cured.
—ANTON CHEKHOV

A treatment trap is when someone is either seriously misdiagnosed or is being treated by a doctor who is more concerned about his or her profits than the patient's well-being. Treatment traps can be deadly.

The book *The Treatment Trap: The Overuse of Medical Care Is Wrecking Your Health and What You Can Do about It* by Rosemary Gibson and Janardan Prasad Singh contains horror stories about treatment traps in America. One of its detailed discussions is about why hospital financial officers are telling doctors to admit one more patient per month—to increase hospital profits, of course. Another is about doctors who perform fake surgeries. Another is about unnecessary CT scans.[48]

Treatment traps are everywhere. One man in California was told he had a life-threatening heart condition he actually did not have. He had triple bypass surgery to "fix" it. Because of the surgery, the man had to give up his job. Two years later, this man and 344 other patients sued Tenet Healthcare, the hospital's owner, as well as eight cardiologists and surgeons who treated them. The defendants ultimately paid $442 million to settle the lawsuits. This is just one of many such instances in the United States.[49]

Consumer Reports listed the ten most overused treatments and tests. These included back surgery, heartburn surgery, prostate treatments, implanted defibrillators, coronary stents, cesarean sections, whole-body scans, high-tech angiographies, high-tech mammograms, and virtual colonoscopies.

If a treatment sounds dubious, it might just be dubious. Ask questions.

The American Association of Retired Persons website provides a great deal more information on this.

(http://www.aarp.org/health/conditions-treatments/info-04-2012/overused-medical-tests-and-treatments.html)

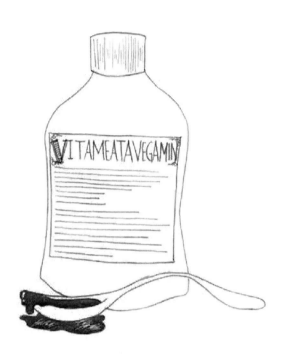

CHAPTER 21

DON'T TAKE MULTIVITAMINS

Food is an important part of a balanced diet.
—Fran Lebowitz

E at a healthy diet, including fresh fruits and vegetables—and forget about the multivitamins, unless prescribed by a doctor.

Evidence against multivitamins, especially those that include vitamin E, is mounting. A study published in 2005 in the *Annals of Internal Medicine* reported that supplemental vitamin E increased mortality. Also that year, a study of people with vascular disease or diabetes found that vitamin E increased the risk of heart failure. In 2011, a study published in the *Journal of the American Medical Association* tied vitamin E supplements to an increased risk of prostate cancer.

Similarly, in 2004, a review of fourteen randomized medical trials found that supplemental vitamins A, C, E, and beta-carotene and the mineral selenium increased mortality.[50] And in 1994, the *New England Journal of Medicine* published a study about Finnish men, all smokers, who had been given daily vitamin E, beta-carotene, both, or a placebo. The study found that those who had taken beta-carotene for five to eight years were more likely to die from lung cancer or heart disease than those who did not.

Two years later, the same journal published another study on vitamin supplements. In this study, people at an increased risk of lung cancer because of asbestos exposure or smoking received either a combination of vitamin A and beta-carotene or a placebo. Investigators stopped the study when they found the risk of death from lung cancer for those who took the vitamins was 46 percent higher![51]

By the way—who wants to choke down a fistful of vitamins every day anyway? Ugh!

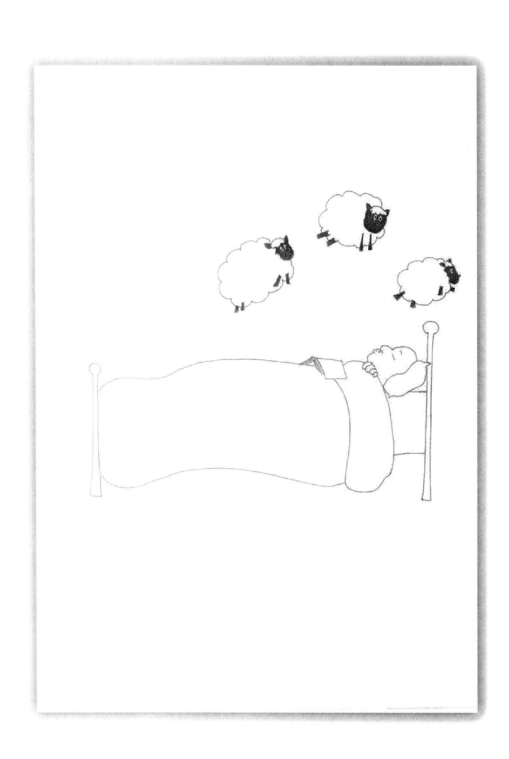

CHAPTER 22

GET A GOOD NIGHT'S SLEEP

Laugh and the world laughs with you, snore and you sleep alone.
—ANTHONY BURGESS

The importance of sleep cannot be overrated. Bad stuff happens if you don't get enough sleep.

According to the World Health Organization, too little sleep leads to higher cancer rates, heart disease, accidents at work, and marital problems. Lack of proper sleep has been associated with a wide variety of social problems, including child abuse, child neglect, more alcohol consumption, binge eating, obesity, blood-pressure problems, and diabetes. All this can stem from a shortage of melatonin and estrogen, which accompany lack of sleep.[52]

Watching the news or exciting movies before going to bed tends to interfere with sleep. It stimulates your brain. Have you ever noticed that your mind is still going strong when you do this? You want your brain to slow down in anticipation of sleep.

Most of us have found a relationship between reading and sleepiness through experience. For many, this started when we were in school. Reading helps most people go to sleep, since it requires your brain to absorb and translate information into meaning, which tires your brain. Reading also tires your eyes. Try reading before bed. You will likely fall asleep faster and get better sleep.

You can try this book at bedtime for starters. If that doesn't work, try your high school physics book—it's sure to work.

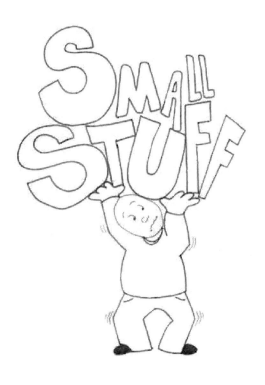

CHAPTER 23

KEEP CONTROL, AND DON'T SWEAT THE SMALL STUFF

> *Don't sweat the small stuff…and it's all small stuff.*
> —RICHARD CARLSON

Wise people know you should just not sweat the small stuff. Life's too short. One trait of stressed-out people is getting into a trap of worrying about trivial things.

Richard Carlson, PhD, and his wife, Kristine Carlson, have sold twenty-five million books around the world. Their advice in these books about how to live a happier, more peaceful, and more respectful life cannot be replicated here. Try reading *Don't Sweat the Small Stuff…and It's All Small Stuff: Simple Ways to Keep the Little Things From Taking Over Your Life* before bed.

Many people already know that high stress levels take a toll on your health. What many people do not realize is that moderate levels of stress, even the smallest hassles, can also take a toll. Research in Switzerland has shown that these small stressors can raise cortisol levels. That's not good. These small stressors can increase the risk of heart disease and weaken the immune system. They can also compromise some types of memory and learning.[53]

An article on CNN.com suggests that we think of the brain as a seesaw. On one side are the frontal lobes, responsible for reasoning. On the other side of the seesaw is the part of the brain called the amygdala, where good and bad emotions are generated. Each person has an internal balance. The balance is hard to maintain because of stress events.[54]

An interesting article in the *Journal of Behavior Therapy and Experimental Psychiatry* told the story of women who were asked to engage in drawing imagery and writing exercises. The women sustained optimism by describing a pleasant or utopian future.

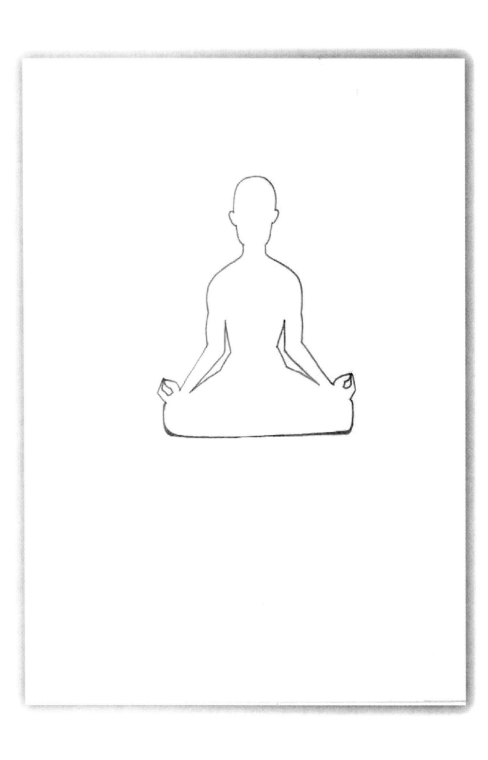

CHAPTER 24

PRAY OR MEDITATE DAILY

*Prayer is when you talk to God. Meditation
is when you're listening.*
—KELSEY GRAMMER

Prayer and meditation are similar. Prayer can create an environment of optimism and a healthy dose of hope. It can also help
people focus and see the bigger picture. It may help people feel
more forgiving and secure. Meditation, including repeating a series
of meaningful, positive, uplifting, and thankful phrases, can retrain
your brain to be more positive, aware, and better able to focus and
let go of unwanted thoughts.[55]

Meditation lowers stress. Research published in 2014 in *Health
Psychology* shows that mindfulness, or meditation, is not only associated with feeling less stressed, it's also linked with decreases in the
stress hormone cortisol.[56]

When you meditate or pray, you clear away the information
overload that builds up every day and contributes to your stress. The
emotional benefits include gaining a new perspective on stressful
situations, building stress-management skills, increasing self-aware-
ness, focusing on the present, and reducing negative emotions.

Meditation can also reduce the incidence of medical problems
such as anxiety disorders, asthma, cancer, depression, heart disease,
high blood pressure, pain, and sleep problems.[57]

Meditating at bedtime can also help you get to sleep.

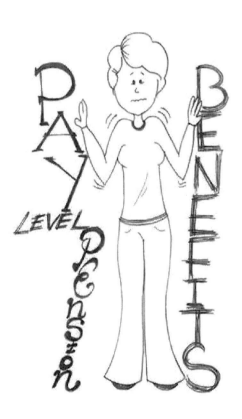

CHAPTER 25

ENVY IS A KILLER

Envy is the art of counting the other fellow's blessings instead of your own.
—HAROLD COFFIN

E nvy can seriously harm your health.[58] Envious people feel hostile, resentful, angry, and irritable. They seldom feel grateful. Envy is related to depression, anxiety, prejudices, and personal unhappiness.

Each of those mental states can impact your health. In addition, envious people are often stressed, overwhelmed, and unpleasant to be around. As a result, envious people may have fewer friends.

Envy involves being upset about what others have. There's no rivalry. Instead, envious people just want what someone else has.

Research by Drs. Richard H. Smith and Sung Hee Kim referred to envy as a painful blend of inferiority, hostility, and resentment that can be both mentally and physically destructive.[59]

The opposite of envy is contentment. Contentment is also a key to a good life. Enjoy what you have, and it will make you happier and healthier.

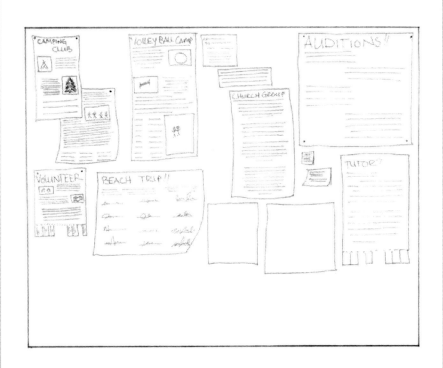

CHAPTER 26

BEING SOCIALLY ACTIVE IS GOOD FOR YOUR HEALTH

Being in control of your life and having realistic expectations about your day-to-day challenges are the keys to stress management—perhaps the most important ingredient to living a happy, healthy and rewarding life.
—MARILU HENNER

People who have satisfying relationships with family, friends, and their community are happier. Dozens of studies have shown that. They also have fewer health problems and live longer.

One study found that lack of strong relationships increased the risk of premature death from all causes by 50 percent—an effect roughly comparable to smoking up to fifteen cigarettes a day.[60]

Having a strong social network can relieve harmful stress. In particular, caring behaviors can trigger the release of stress-reducing hormones.

Depression and social isolation affect one in seven people over sixty-five years of age. In addition, social isolation adversely affects long-term health. On the other hand, leisure activities and social interaction contribute to improved health in older adults.[61]

A study showed a wide range of responses (both physical and emotional) when engaged in social activities. These included increased alertness, social activity, self-worth, optimism about life, and positive changes in health behavior.[62]

The bottom line here is that everyone needs social interaction—so get out and have some. You can easily find people with whom to interact in religious, social, civic, and educational organizations.

A good start may be to invite neighbors over for dinner. Tom's secret favorite is hot dogs and boiled potatoes--but I'm not advocating that as a menu you should serve to new friends.

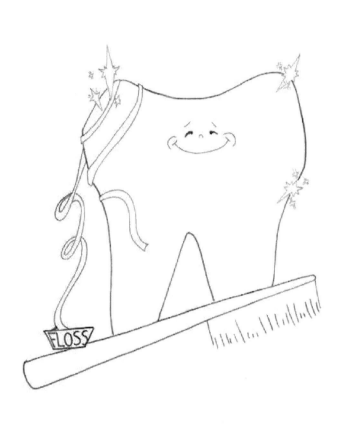

CHAPTER 27

BRUSH AND FLOSS YOUR
TEETH REGULARLY

*We idolized the Beatles, except for those of us who
idolized the Rolling Stones, who in those days
still had many of their original teeth.*
—DAVE BARRY

Poor oral hygiene can lead to serious health problems. A study at Bristol University in England has discovered that a common bacterium responsible for tooth decay and gum disease can break out into the bloodstream and lead to heart disease and blood clots.[63]

The Mayo Clinic reported the same thing, noting that many medical issues, including endocarditis, cardiovascular disease, premature birth, low birth weight, diabetes, and osteoporosis can all be linked to poor dental hygiene.[64]

The human mouth harbors a lot of wildlife in the form of over six hundred types of living bacteria, many of which can damage your overall health. Brushing your teeth regularly and remembering to floss seem like small prices to pay for better health.

Good dental hygiene can result in fewer of your teeth being drilled or pulled and may help you live longer.

Good dental hygiene will also make your breath more pleasant. That might help you make friends, who are also good for your health. Amazing!

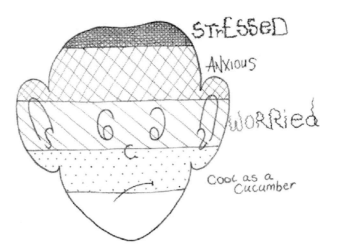

CHAPTER 28

LEARN TO COPE WITH STRESS
IN HEALTHFUL WAYS

If you ask what is the single most important key to longevity,
I would have to say it is avoiding worry, stress and tension.
And if you didn't ask me, I'd still have to say it.
—GEORGE BURNS

According to the American Psychological Association, not only are stress levels increasing but also the ability to cope with stress is decreasing.[65]

Stress can be the root cause of many health problems. A study in 2012 showed that 53 percent of Americans reported personal health problems as a result of stresses, including the following:[66]

- money (75 percent)
- work (70 percent)
- personal health concerns (53 percent)
- job stability (49 percent)
- housing costs (49 percent)
- personal safety (32 percent)
- the economy (67 percent)
- relationships (58 percent)
- family responsibilities (57 percent)
- family health problems (53 percent)

Conversely, the way people cope with stress is important. While eating well and exercising are often noted as stress beaters, only about half the people in a study identified these as major factors. Other things are more important. For instance, each of the following reduces stress:[67]

- good family relationships (76 percent)
- getting enough sleep (60 percent)
- good friendships (60 percent)
- doing well in career or studies (59 percent)

Poor health can cause stress too. This is a destructive loop: poor health leads to stress, which leads to poorer health.

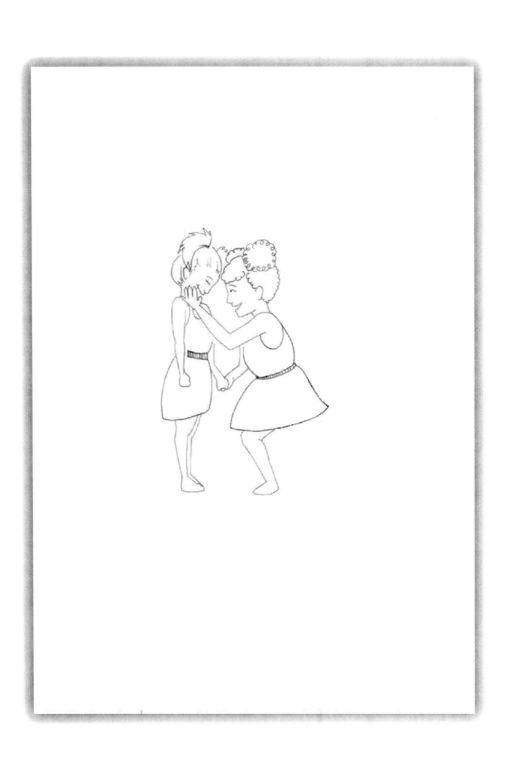

CHAPTER 29

SELF-ESTEEM IS IMPORTANT TO YOUR HEALTH

Wanting to be someone else is a waste of the person you are.
—MARILYN MONROE

Poor self-esteem is bad for your health. Self-esteem can be improved through eating nutritious meals, avoiding cigarettes, drinking plenty of water, exercising, avoiding too much alcohol and other drugs, setting realistic goals, and surrounding yourself with positive-minded people, according to the University of Michigan.[68]

On the last of these, scientists found that relationships and social connections build self-esteem and reduce harmful stress. Similarly, a large study in Sweden concluded that dementia risk was lowest among those who had a variety of satisfying connections with friends and relatives, which helped increase self-esteem.[69] Likewise, according to research at Rush University Medical Center, being socially active may help keep you mentally sharp in old age and improve self-esteem.[70]

Something you're probably noticing by now is that many of the chapters and ideas in this book are linked. Things like good oral hygiene can improve your self-esteem, give you more confidence and—ta-da—improve your social life.

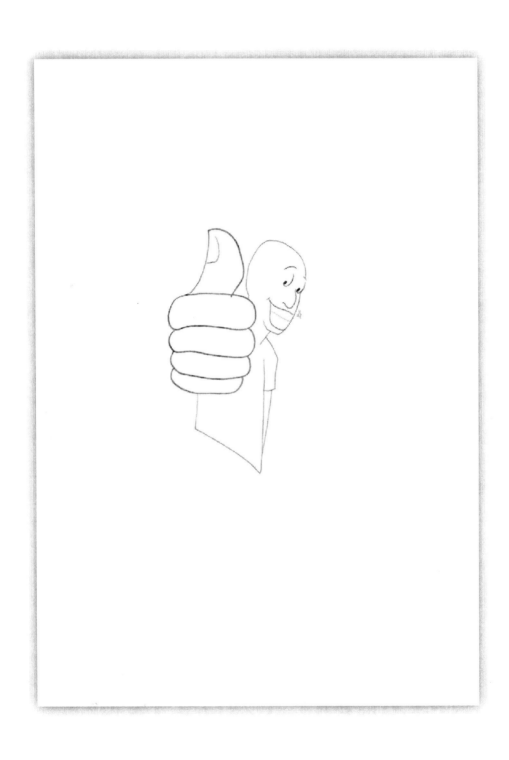

CHAPTER 30

BE RESILIENT

A wise woman wishes to be no one's enemy; a
wise woman refuses to be anyone's victim.
—MAYA ANGELOU

Some people believe modern America is characterized by a "victim mentality." To be considered a victim today is almost faddish in some circles. But it's risky, too.

People with a victim mentality are often self-absorbed, defensive, and stubborn and have a strong sense of learned helplessness— a sense that other people cause their problems. It is a mental illness and a direct cause of mortality and morbidity.[71]

Victims also have trouble holding a job. They are often overweight, pessimistic, and easily depressed, and they have more adverse health events.

Resilience is the capacity to withstand stress and catastrophe. Resilience can save your life. Being resilient doesn't mean life is stress-free. No life is stress-free. Everyone feels grief, sadness, and a range of other emotions after adversity and loss.

Resilient people work through the emotions and effects of stress and painful events, while "victims" do not.[72]

People who are resilient live longer.[73] Healthy people show more optimism and hope in the face of a health challenge. Positive expectations have been shown to predict better health after heart transplants,[74] quicker recovery from coronary bypass surgery, and less severe angina pain, among other medical problems.[75]

Resilience has also been shown to reduce mortality in people with chronic diseases, and it can preserve mental and physical health.[76]

Living in a state of self-pity all the time does not really attract friends.

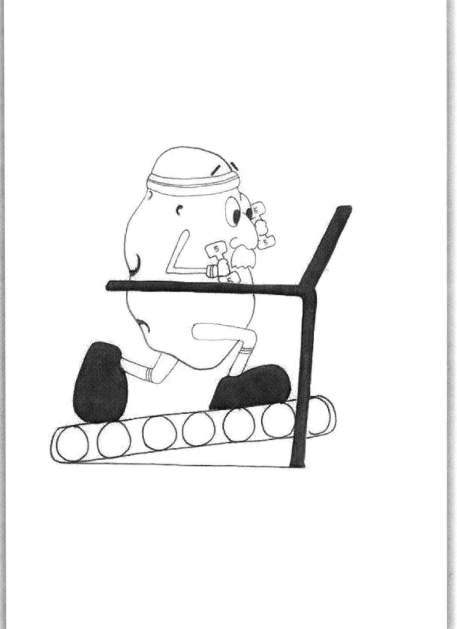

CHAPTER 31

COUCH-POTATO SYNDROME IS DEADLY

An early-morning walk is a blessing for the whole day.
—HENRY DAVID THOREAU

Walking can significantly increase your lifespan. A large meta-study (a study of other studies) showed that walking reduced cardiovascular events and heart-attack deaths by almost one-third.[77]
Walking also reduces the risk of chronic diseases, including:

- high blood pressure
- high cholesterol
- high blood sugar[78]

Walking can help you be in the moment. It can give you time to relax or listen to your favorite music. Walking can help you sleep better and provide you with healthy doses of vitamin D. All the better if you can walk with your dog or a friend.

While some advocate running over walking, that extra expenditure of energy and the wear and tear on your knees may not be necessary from a health perspective.

About eighteen centuries ago, Hippocrates referred to walking as man's best medicine. (Hippocrates knew his stuff, didn't he? He's the guy who told other doctors to quit poisoning people for hire.)

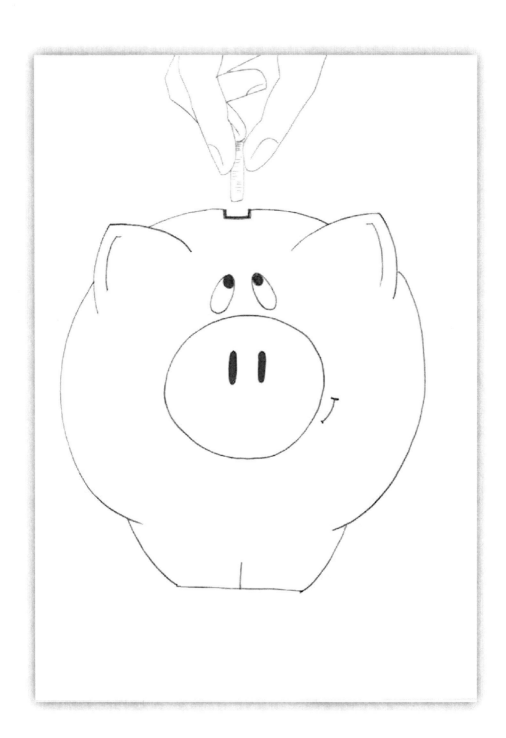

CHAPTER 32

MANAGE YOUR MONEY WELL

*People have got to learn: if they don't have cookies
in the cookie jar, they can't eat cookies.*
—SUZE ORMAN

M oney stresses are bad for your health.
For the majority of Americans, money is a major source of stress. A Harris Poll in August 2014 found that 72 percent of Americans reported feeling stressed about money some of the time during the past month. An additional 22 percent said they experienced extreme stress about money during the past month. This is especially true for parents and younger adults. Virtually everyone in the United States today has money stress.[79]

Money stress has caused people to ignore their health. Nearly one in five Americans say they have either considered skipping or did skip going to the doctor because of financial concerns.[80] A second study showed that such people self-rated their health as worse.[81]

Being economically deprived can cause stress. However, it is not only low-income people who have money problems. The Gallup-Healthways Well-Being Index showed that while emotional well-being increased with income—up to about $75,000 a year in income—it did not continue to improve for people making more than that.

This is another example showing that contentment makes a huge difference.

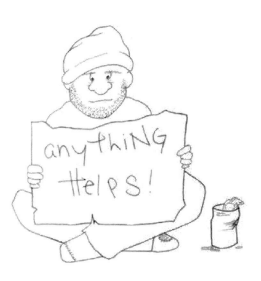

CHAPTER 33

TREAT PEOPLE WITH RESPECT
AND KINDNESS

*Kindness and politeness are not overrated
at all. They're underused.*
—TOMMY LEE JONES

Being kind to others improves your own health and makes you feel better too.

A Harris Interactive study of 3,351 randomly selected people showed that the 76 percent who volunteered said they felt healthier overall. They said helping others helped lower their own stress.[82]

Helping others releases "feel-good" hormones such as serotonin, oxytocin, endorphins, and dopamine. Acts of kindness result in the release of these hormones.[83]

Therefore, do something nice for someone else today. Try paying for the order of someone in line behind you in a drive-through restaurant. They won't have a chance to thank you, and somehow that may make you feel good.

Give bigger-than-expected tips. That means a ton to someone who serves food for a living.

Volunteer to help a charity. Donate something you don't use. Redirecting gifts from yourself to charity will also make you feel good.

Random acts of kindness to strangers can give you a huge boost. Start today.

In many cases, just taking the time to really listen to people will make you feel better. We all need someone to talk to, and sometimes people don't have that in their lives.

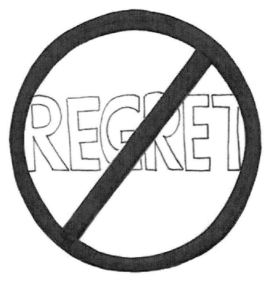

CHAPTER 34

LIVE LIFE TO HAVE FEW REGRETS

*Finish each day and be done with it. You have done what
you could. Some blunders and absurdities no doubt crept in;
forget them as soon as you can. Tomorrow is a new day.*
—RALPH WALDO EMERSON

Rule number one is to avoid doing things you're going to regret later.

Rule number two is don't hold on to grudges.

Rule number three is don't keep putting something off that you have wanted to do all your life. You may wake up someday and realize it's too late.

Those are the kinds of things regrets are made of.

Life's Little Instruction Book by H. Jackson Brown has sold over nine million copies and been translated into thirty-three languages. Among the notable observations from his book is: "Twenty years from now you will be more disappointed by the things you didn't do than by the ones you did do."

James Clear wrote in *The #1 Regret of Dying People* that too many people spend the last days of their lives regretting things they did when they were younger. Brown's advice would be "live a good, honorable life which you can enjoy a second time when you are old."

Far too many people end up at the final stages of life regretting things that they did or did not do.

It's not too late to start following rules one, two, and three.

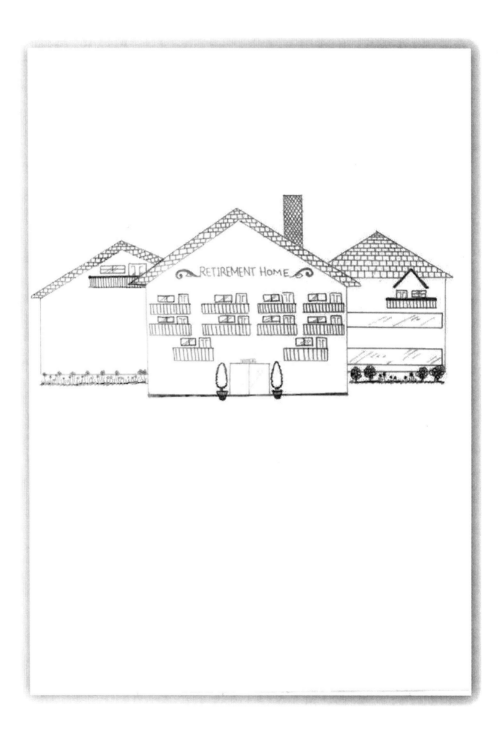

CHAPTER 35

RETIREMENT CAN BE BAD
FOR YOUR HEALTH

Half our life is spent trying to find something to do with
the time we have rushed through life trying to save.
—WILL ROGERS

Everyone talks about how much they will enjoy retirement. Ah, the leisure of it all! People envision whole days of sitting around and doing nothing.

The facts suggest that idleness is really quite bad for your health.[84] Retirement increases the probability of suffering from clinical depression. It also lowers the likelihood of being in "good or excellent" health by 40 percent.[85]

Retirement also increases problems with mobility and daily activities by 5 to 16 percent.[86] A study of sixteen thousand Greeks in 2007 reported that retirees were 51 percent more likely to die than people working at the same age. All of us have known people who died shortly after retirement. A friend of ours always said that they were dying of boredom. Studies have shown this is at least partially true.

A study at Shell Oil in 2005 showed that early retirees engage in unhealthy behaviors more often. These include heavy drinking, smoking, and adopting an unhealthy diet (combined with less exercise). The study found that people who retire at fifty-five are

89 percent more likely to die in the ten years after retirement than those who retire at sixty-five.[87]

When you retire, you need to find useful things to do. The leisure activities you enjoy during your preretirement years may have been fun because they were rare. If those same activities are all you have to do, they can become dull fairly fast.

Try volunteering. One of America's most noted agronomy scientists stayed busy in his elder years by volunteering at a hospital

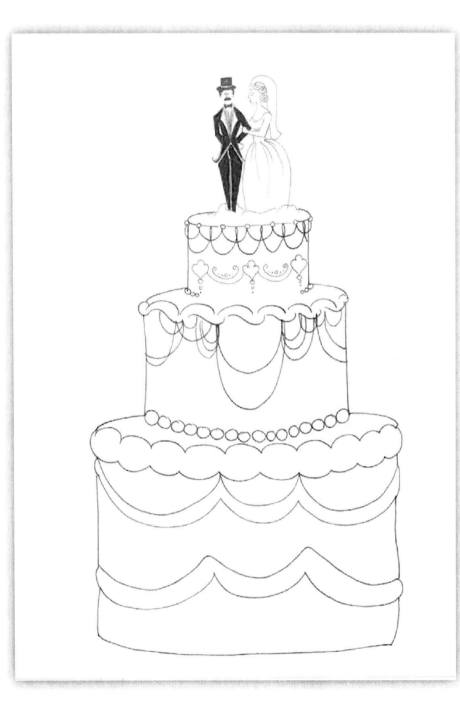

CHAPTER 36

GENETICS IS A BIG DEAL

Raising kids is part joy and part guerrilla warfare.
—ED ASNER

G enetics play a role in longevity. But making good choices in life can make a huge difference. This book is about choices you can make. It's important to know the risks you may inherit and advise your doctor of them.

A partial list of inheritable traits include vision problems, eczema, migraines, irritable bowel syndrome, allergies, attention deficit hyperactivity disorder, anxiety disorders, breast cancer, depression and bipolar disorders, obsessive-compulsive disorders, cystic fibrosis, sickle-cell anemia, hemophilia, and heart disease.[88]

Alas, this is only a short list of potential genetic disorders. If you want to see other medical conditions that can be inherited, look up "genetic disorders" on Wikipedia.[89] Be ready to read multiple pages of information.

You need to be aware of your family history, especially about what family members died of and at what age. That kind of history can be useful in considering the type and frequency of doctor screenings. If scary diseases run in your family or your wife or husband's, be sure to share that with your own children at the right time. The right time is not during childhood. Let them enjoy being children.

Know your family health history and take actions to address these issues before they become a problem.[90]

Warning: digging into family history can turn up some dead relatives you may not take great pride in knowing about. One person Tom knows dug into his family tree and discovered an ancestor who fought in the Revolutionary War--as a German mercenary.

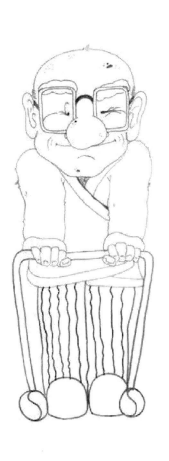

CHAPTER 37

IF YOU LIVE LONG ENOUGH, YOU ARE GOING TO GET OLD

Age is a matter of mind, if you don't mind, it doesn't matter.
—BETSEY JOHNSON

Aging is relative. On his eightieth birthday, someone asked Oliver Wendell Holmes to share his birthday wish. He is said to have replied, "Ah, to be seventy again."

Aging starts the day you're born. It's really not a bad thing. Many people feel more relaxed and calm and peaceful as they age.

Aging is a journey. You may as well enjoy it. There's nothing you can do to stop it anyway.

In a way, aging is an adventure. If you embrace it and are emotionally prepared to enjoy each new stage, what could be better?

People are living longer. In 1880, the average life expectancy was fifty. By 1900, the average was about fifty-two. By 1920, it was sixty-two. By 1950, it was sixty-five. By 1970, the average life expectancy was 70.8 years. In 2008, life expectancy was 78.0 years.[91] Life expectancy in 2020 is projected to be 82.93.[92]

The Mayo Clinic suggests a good way to live longer is to eat a healthy diet, exercise regularly, and avoid too much sun. It's that simple.[93] The Mayo Clinic also noted most anti-aging creams and pills simply don't work—and they may cause other medical problems.

Our suggestion is to read this book carefully and follow the guidelines. We also strongly recommend giving this book to all your friends and relatives. Okay, you may put that last sentence in the category of crass commercialism, but authors have to eat, too.

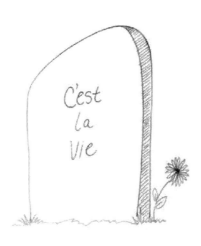

CHAPTER 38

DYING IS PART OF LIFE

Age is not a particularly interesting subject. Anyone can get old. All you have to do is live long enough.
—GROUCHO MARX

A good goal is to age gracefully and when the time comes die with dignity. Who really wants to be in a miserable treatment trap of endless medical care and procedures?

So what if you gain a few days lying around in some hospital? Is adding a few more days to your life really important to you at the end?

Given the option, wouldn't most people rather be at home in their final days with those who love them than be in an intensive care unit with tubes galore and a machine helping them breathe?

We, the authors of this book, would much rather die at home than after miserable days or weeks in an intensive care unit.

Make sure your wishes are known to your family, especially your adult children. Create an advanced directive to help your family make important decisions about your health and final days.

Didn't someone once say that death is life's last great adventure? We hear you…it sounds like "phonus balonus" to the authors, too. Phonus balonus is genuine slang from the 1920s. It means "nonsense" but sounds better.

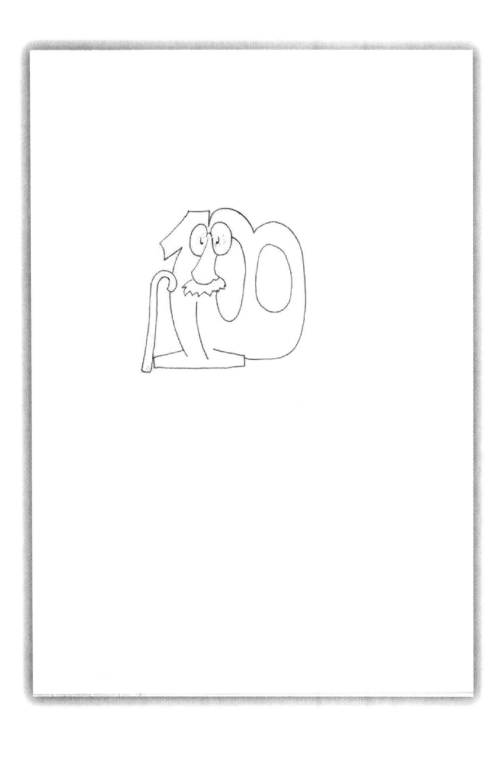

CHAPTER 39

WHO WANTS TO LIVE TO BE A HUNDRED?

> *Life should not be a journey to the grave with the intention of*
> *arriving safely in a pretty and well preserved body, but rather*
> *to skid in broadside in a cloud of smoke, thoroughly used up,*
> *totally worn out, and loudly proclaiming—Wow! What a Ride!*
> —HUNTER S. THOMPSON

A re you sure you want to live to be one hundred?

Aging and dying are part of life. Only about fifty-five thousand living Americans are over one hundred years old. Sadly, the average income of these people is quite low. The average income of women and men over one hundred is $12,200 and $17,500, respectively. Four-fifths of the centenarians in the United States are women. Therefore, most centenarians are living with incomes only slightly above the poverty level of $11,670. People who live to be one hundred have simply outlived their retirement savings and their ability to be independent.[94]

One of the authors previously lived next door to a ninety-eight-year-old woman. One day she called and asked if we and our kids could come over to help her with something. She wanted us to call her by her first name. That's all. She explained she had outlived all of her contemporaries and sadly never heard her first name spoken anymore. It made us feel good to do that for her.

We all aspire to live a long and happy life. However, we will all pass away in time.

Try to enjoy your life as much as possible and worry less about how and when you'll die. One thing is certain: When that time comes, no one will ever look back and wish they'd spent more time at work.

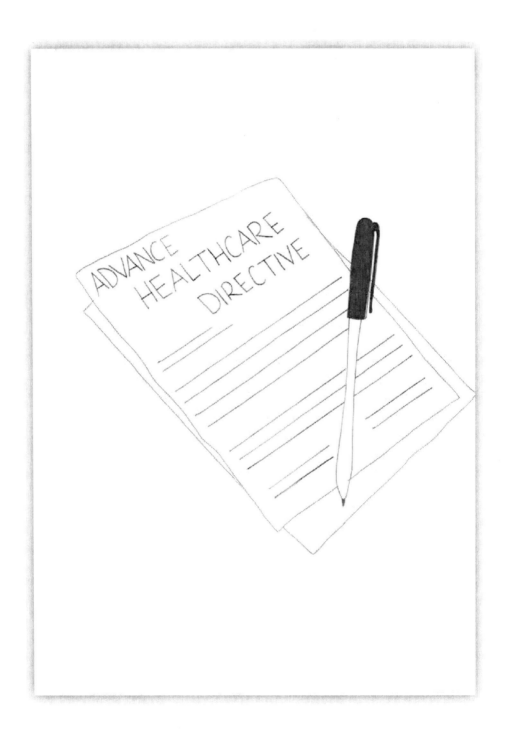

CHAPTER 40

CREATE AN ADVANCED DIRECTIVE

Failing to plan is planning to fail.
—ALAN LAKEIN

News flash: You are going to die someday. So is everyone else. Nobody gets out alive. You may as well accept that fact and prepare for it.

One of the best things you can do for your family is to create an advanced directive. An advance directive tells providers what to do if you are unable to make decisions.

Do you want to be put on dialysis or breathing machines? Should you be resuscitated if your heart stops? Should you be on a feeding tube if it comes to that? Do you want to donate your organs? Normally, your physician decides whether you are capable of making these decisions. In some states, the opinions of two physicians are required, one to confirm the other.

All medical personnel except emergency-care providers must follow your advanced directive. Emergency medical personnel (ambulance, emergency room, etc.) must do what is necessary to stabilize a patient.

The 1990 Patient Self-Determination Act (PSDA) encourages everyone to decide now about the types and extent of medical care they want to accept or refuse if they become unable to make those decisions later. PSDA also requires all health-care agencies to recognize a living will and durable power of attorney for health care. The act applies to hospitals, long-term care facilities, and home health agencies that get Medicare and Medicaid reimbursement.

An advanced directive will greatly benefit your family. When you are seriously ill, and perhaps near the end of your life, relatives will experience great stress. Don't force them to make life-or-death decisions for you. Recently, the mother-in-law of a friend of ours was near the end. The closer it came, the more the family members argued about what kind of health care their mother should continue to receive. Not having an advanced directive forced siblings to argue with one another. That's not what anyone wants.

EPILOGUE

You have choices. It's never too late. The introduction to this book said you will learn what choices you can make to lead a healthier and happier life. As you've read, health and happiness are inextricably linked. It's hard to be happy if you're sick, and it's hard to be healthy if you're miserable. Well-being is the opposite of misery.

The goal of this book is to empower readers to take control of their own health and well-being. Key determinants of your health and well-being include enjoyment of life, contentment, good relationships with friends and family, having a job you can tolerate or even teach yourself to enjoy, being an active member of your community, contributing to the welfare of others, and having good goals.

You have a huge number of health risk factors—a hundred or so, in fact. If one aspect of your health seems good, but the other ninety-nine are out of sync, you're probably going to lead an unhappy and unhealthy life. No medical "treatment" will ever be available to cover all of your risk factors.

Job satisfaction is huge. You've probably noticed how your risk factors are interactive. If you're unhappy with most aspects of your life, you probably are not going to make the best of your job.

Grudges, hatred, jealousy, and envy will poison and embitter you from the inside out. You have choices and options. You don't have to live like that.

Don't wait for someone else to come to you to bury the hatchet, even if they started the mess. You may have a long wait.

Life's not fair. So what? If you spend your life waiting for fairness to be handed to you, be prepared for a life of disappointment. Instead, acknowledge that life is not fair and go about making the most of it.

If your childhood was not perfect (and whose ever was?), so what? You're an adult now. Get over it. Make up for it by loving your children and grandchildren with abandon. The rewards will be endless if you give them the childhood you wish you had.

Someday, many of us will be wheeled into a hospice or nursing home. When that happens, you may have time to reflect on your life. You likely won't remember any pay raise you got, the fancy car you once had, or even how nice your home was. But at that moment, the respect of your family and friends will be huge in your life.

At the risk of sounding like authors who can't resist writing about the same thing again, people will never wish they had spent more time watching television or playing video games, nor will people on their deathbeds take pride in winning lots of arguments with their spouses.

It is the good times and the good things one does that make life livable. Hopefully, those are the things we will remember in the end.

Finally, we pick on physicians a bit in this book. Some deserve it. But hats off to the doctors who work with each patient to determine the desirable outcome and then use the safest, least invasive, least medicated way to achieve it.

Notes

1. Elahe Izadi, "Using a Public Restroom Hand Dryer? You May Be Spreading Bacteria All Over the Place." *Washington Post*, November 21, 2014.

2. Edyta Margas, Emma Maguire, Carolyn R. Berland, Francis Welander, and John Holah, Assessment of the environmental microbiological cross contamination following hand drying with paper hand towels or an air blade dryer, *Journal of Applied Microbiology*, (2013) 115: 572–82. doi:10.1111/jam.12248.

3. Chandler Smith, "Gallup Poll: 70% of Americans Hate Their Stupid Jobs." *RYOT News+Action*, accessed February 20, 2015, http://www.ryot.org/gallup-poll-70-americans-disengaged-jobs/376177.

4. Alexander Kjerulf. "5 Ways Hating Your Job Can Ruin Your Health (According to Science)," *Huffington Post Healthy Living 9 (blog)*. March 26, 2014, http://www.huffingtonpost.com/alexander-kjerulf/happiness-tips_b_5001073.html.

5. "The Effect of Hate on Children," Canadian Counseling and Psychotherapy Association, accessed February 27, 2015. http://www.ccpa-accp.ca/blog/?p=2454.

6. Dan Pink. "The Puzzle of Motivation," accessed March 1, 2015. http://www.ted.com/talks/dan_pink_on_motivation?language=en.

7. "Fad Diets." University of Pittsburgh Medical Center, accessed March 2, 2015, http://www.upmc.com/patients-visitors/education/nutrition/pages/fad-diets.aspx.

8. Jeanie Lerce Davis, "Diabetes and the Risk of Fad Diets," WebMD, accessed February 28, 2014, http://www.webmd.com/diabetes/features/diabetes-risk-fad-diets.

9. Julie Beck, "It's Probably Best to Avoid Antibacterial Soaps." WebMD, accessed February 26, 2015. http://www.theatlantic.com/health/archive/2014/08/its-probably-best-to-avoid-antibacterial-soaps/375899/.

10. Matthew Hoffman, "Antibacterial Soap: Do You Need It to Keep Your Home Clean?" WebMD, accessed March 2, 2015, http://www.webmd.com/health-ehome-9/antibacterial-soap-cleaners.

11. Lisa Baertlein, "When Should You See a Doctor for a Cold?" accessed March 3, 2015, http://www.everydayhealth.com.

12. "Generic Drugs: Questions and Answers." US Food and Drug Administration, accessed March 2, 2015. http://www.fda.gov/drugs/resourcesforconsumers.

13. Patrick J. Skerrett, "Generic Drugs, Don't Ask, Don't Tell," *Harvard Health* (blog), January 7, 2013, http://www.health.harvard.edu/blog/generic-drugs-dont-ask-just-tell-201301075768.

14. "Over the Counter Medications: Use in General and Special Populations, Therapeutic Errors, Misuse, Storage and Disposal," American College of Preventive Medicine, accessed March 5, 2015. http://c.ymcdn.com/sites/www.acpm.org/resource/resmgr/timetools-files/otcmedsclinicalreference.pdf.

15. Scott Gavura, "Dr. Oz and the Terrible, Horrible, No Good, Very Bad Day, "Science Based Medicine, accessed March

17, 2015, http://www.sciencebasedmedicine.org/dr-oz-and-the-terrible-horrible-no-good-very-bad-day.

16. Mayo Clinic Staff. "Red Wine and Resveratrol: Good for Your Heart?" Mayo Clinic, accessed March 16, 2015, http://mayoclinic.org/diseases-conditions/heart-disease/in-depth/red-wine/art-20048281.

17. Raquel Maurier, "Resveratrol May Be a Natural Exercise Performance Enhancer: U of A Medical Research, accessed January 20, 2015, http://www.ualberta.ca/news/3023/june/resveratrolmaybeanaturalexerciseperformanceenhabceruafamedicalresearch.

18. A.L. Klatsky and Gerald D. Friedman, "Alcohol and Longevity," *American Journal of Public Health* 85, no. 1 (1995), accessed February 23, 2015, http://www.ncbi.nlm.nih.gov/pmc/articles/PMC1614277/2015.

19. PBS, *9 Ways Humor Heals*.

20. William Fry, "The Connection between Laughter, Humor, and Good Health," accessed February 27, 2015, http://www2.ca.uky.edu/hes/fcs/factshts/hsw-caw-807.pdf.

21. Jonathan Petre, "You Really Can Be Bored to Death, "*Daily Mail*, accessed March 1, 2015, http://www.dailymail.co.uk/sciencetech/article-1249073/You-really-bored-death-scientists-discover.html#ixzz3TDXITG3K.

22. Scott Edwards, "Humor, Laughter, and Those Aha Moments," *On the Brain: The Harvard Mahoney Neuroscience Institute Letter*

16, no. 2, accessed February 19, 2015, http://hms.harvard.edu/sites/default/files/HMS_OTB_Spring10_Vol16_No2.pdf.

23. Leo Babauta, "5 Powerful Reasons to Eat Slower," *Zen Habits*, accessed March 3, 2015, http://zenhabits.net/5-powerful-reasons-to-eat-slower.

24. Brian St. Pierre, "All about Eating Slowly," Precision Nutrition, accessed February 24, 2015, http://www.precisionnutrition.com/all-about-slow-eating.

25. Jane E. Brody, "Babies Know: A Little Dirt Is Good for You," *New York Times*, January 27, 2009, www.nytimes.com/2009/01/27/health/27brod.html?_r=0.

26. Megan Scudellari, "Let Them Eat Dirt: Early Exposure to Microbes Shapes the Mammalian Immune System by Subduing Inflammatory T Cells," *The Scientist*, March 22, 2012.

27. Richard West, Russell Meserve, and Kevin Stanovich, "Cognitive Sophistication Does Not Attenuate the Bias Blind Spot," accessed March 5, 2015, http://psycnet.apa.org/psycinfo/2012-14753-001.

28. "7 Benefits of Having a Hobby," Positively Present, accessed April 1, 2015. http://www.positivelypresent.com/2013/06/benefits-of-having-a-hobby.html.

29. Rachel Hanson, "Ten Hobbies for Retirees," accessed April 1, 2015, http://seniors.lovetoknow.com/Ten_Hobbies_for_Retirees.

30. Lynne Giles, Gary Glonek, Mary Luszcz, and Gary Andrews. "Effect of Social Networks on 10 Year Survival in Very Old

Australians: The Australian Longitudinal Study of Aging," *Journal of Epidemiology & Community Health*. 2005, accessed February 15, 2015. http://jech.bmj.com/content/59/7/574.abstract?maxtoshow=&HITS=10&hits=10&

31. Anthony Paika and Kenneth Sanchagrina. "Social Isolation in America, An Artifact," *American Sociological Review*, 2013, accessed February 27, 2015, http://asr.sagepub.com/content/early/2013/04/05/0003122413482919.abstract.

32. Candyce Kroenke, Laura Kibzansky, Eva Schernhammer, Michelle Holmes, and Ichiro Kawachi, "Social Networks, Social Support, and Survival after Breast Cancer Diagnosis," 2006, accessed February 27, 2015. http://jco.ascopubs.org/content/24/7/1105.full.pdf.

33. Nicholas Christakis and James Fowler, "The Spread of Obesity in a Large Social Network over 32 Years," *New England Journal of Medicine*. 2007, accessed February 26, 2015. http://www.nejm/org/doi/full/10.1056/NEJMsa066082.

34. Kristina Orth-Gomer, Annika Rosengen, and Lars Wilhelmsen, "Lack of Social Support and Incidence of Coronary Heart Disease in Middle-Aged Swedish Men," *Psychosomatic Medicine* 55, no. 1 (2015), accessed March 2, 2015. http://www.researchgate.net/publication/14752050_Lack_of_social_support_and_incidence_of_coronary_heart_disease_in_middle-aged_Swedish_men.

35. Steve Bradt, "Wandering Mind Not a Happy Mind," *Harvard Gazette*, 2010, accessed March 6, 2015, http://news.harvard.edu/gazette/story/2010/11/wandering-mind-not-a-happy-mind/Archives of Internal Medicine.

36. Kathleen Dohemy, "7 Dangerous Drug Mistakes," 2013, accessed February 15, 2015, http://www.webmd.com/a-to-z-guides/features/7-dangerous-drug-mistakes?page=4.

37. Robert Blendon, John Benson, and Joachim Hero, "Public Trust in Physicians—US. Medicine in International Perspective,"*New England Journal of Medicine*, 2014, accessed February 24, 2015. http://www.nejm.org/doi/full/10.1056/NEJMp1407373.

38. Peter Ubel, "Why Don't Americans Trust Doctors?" *Forbes*, 2014, accessed April 4, 2015, http://www.forbes.com/sites/peterubel/2014/12/19/why-dont-americans-trust-doctors.

39. Velma L. Payne, Hardeep Singh, Ashley N.D. Meyer, Lewis Levy, David Harrison, and Mark L. Graber. "Patient-Initiated Second Opinions: Systematic Review of the Characteristics and Impact on Diagnosis, Treatment, and Satisfaction," Mayo Clinic Proceedings, 2014, accessed February 17, 2015, http://www.mayoclinicproceedings.org/article/S0025-6196%2814%2900245-6/fulltext.

40. Peter Eisler and Barbara Hansen, "Doctors Perform Thousands of Unnecessary Surgeries," 2013, accessed March 27, 2015. http://www.usatoday.com/story/news/nation/2013/06/18/unnecessary-surgery-usa-today-investigation/2435009.

41. The hospital-safety scoreboard can be accessed at http://www.hospitalsafetyscore.org.

42. Deborah Kotz, "Overmedication: Are Americans Taking Too Many Drugs?" 2010, accessed February 22, 2015, http://health.usnews.com/health-news/managing-your-healthcare/

diabetes/articles/2010/10/07/overmedication-are-americans-taking-too-many-drugs.

43. "Safe Use Initiative Fact Sheet," US Food and Drug Administration, 2014, accessed February 12, 2015, http://www.fda.gov/Drugs/DrugSafety/ucm188760.htm.

44. "Medication Errors," Agency for Healthcare Research and Quality, 2013, accessed March 6, 2015, http://psnet.ahrq.gov/primer.aspx?primerID=23.

45. Siri Carpenter, "The Epidemic of Overmedication," *NBC News*, 2008, accessed February 27, 2015, http://www.nbcnews.com/id/27645077/ns/health-health_care/t/epidemic-overmedica-tion/#.VSL4-rpjoQ5.

46. Alan Schwarz. "Thousands of Toddlers Are Medicated for A.D.H.D., Report Finds, Raising Worries," *New York Times* online, May 17, 2014, http://www.nytimes.com/2014/05/17/us/among-experts-scrutiny-of-attention-disorder-diagnoses-in-2-and-3-year-olds.html?_r=0.

47. Ibid.

48. Rosemary Gibson and Janardan Prasad Singh, *The Treatment Trap: How the Overuse of Medical Care Is Wrecking Your Health and What You Can Do to Prevent It* (Lanham: Maryland Ivan R. Dee), 2010.

49. "Treatment Traps to Avoid," ConsumerReports.org, 2007, accessed April 20, 2015, http://www.consumerreports.org/cro/2012/08/treatment-traps-to-avoid/index.htm.

50 Goran Bjelakovic, Desaslava Nikolova, Lise Lott Gluud, Rosa G. Simonetti, and Christian Gluud. "Antioxidant Supplements for Prevention of Mortality in Healthy Participants and Patients with Various Diseases," Cochrane Database of Systematic Reviews 14, no. 3, accessed March 9, 2015.

51. Paul Offit, "Don't Take Your Vitamins, "*New York Times* online, June 9, 2013, http://www.nytimes.com/2013/06/09/opinion/sunday/dont-take-your-vitamins.html.

52. Robert H. Woods. "Your Night Shift Job Is Killing You" (presentation, Hospitality Summit Conference, Las Vegas, NV, 2010).

53. Carmen and Jozsef Haller. "Stress and the Social Brain: Behavioural Effects and Neurobiological Mechanisms," *Nature* online, April 20, 2015, http://www.nature.com/nrn/journal/v16/n5/full/nrn3918.html.

54. Joanne Chen, "How to Stop Sweating the Small Stuff," CNN. coma, accessed April 1, 2015, http://www.cnn.com/2014/01/13/living/sweat-small-stuff-real-simple.

55. Roya R. Rad, "The Positive Psychological Effects of Prayer," HuffPost Healthy Living (blog), April 11, 2013, http://www.huffingtonpost.com/roya-r-rad-ma-psyd/prayer_b_3055127.html.

56. "Mindfulness Meditation Could Lower Levels Of Cortisol, The Stress Hormone," Huffington Post Healthy Living (blog), March 31, 2013.

57. Sian Beilock, "How Mindfulness Medication Alters the Brain," Choke (blog), *Psychology Today*, June 3, 2011, https://www.psychologytoday.com/blog/choke/201106/how-mindfulness-meditation-alters-the-brain.

58. "Seven Deadly Sins," accessed March 17, 2015, http://www. newworldencyclopedia.org/entry/Seven_Deadly_Sins.

59. Richard Smith and Sung Hee Kim, "Comprehending Envy," *Psychological Bulletin* 133, no. 1 (2007).

60. Mark Crowley, "The Sharp Drop-off in Worker Happiness— And What Your Company Can Do About It," *Fast Company*, April 30, 2012, accessed March 30, 2015, http"//www.fastcompany.com/1835578/sharp-drop-worker-happiness-and-what-your-company-can-do-about-it.

61. Po-Ju Chang, Linda Wray, and Yeqiang Lin, "Social Relationships, Leisure Activity and Health in Older Adults," *Health Psychology* 33, no. 6 (2014).

62. Colin Greaves and Lou Farbus, "Effects of Creative and Social Activity on the Health and Well-Being of Socially Isolated Older People: Outcomes from a Multi-Method Observational Study," *Perspectives on Health*, 2013.

63. Stephen Adams, "Why Not Brushing Your Teeth Can Kill You," *Telegraph*, September 6, 2010.

64. Martha Grogan, "Will Taking Care of My Teeth Help Prevent Heart Disease?" Mayo Clinic, accessed March 17, 2015, http://mayoclinic.org/healthy-lifestyle/adult-health/expert-answers/heart-disease-prevention/faq-20057986.

65. American Psychological Association, "Stress in America™ 2012 Highlights: Missing the Healthcare Connection," 2012, accessed February 26, 2015. http://www.apa.org/news/press/releases/stress/2012/report-summary.aspx.

66. Ibid.

67. American Psychological Association: Adults' Stress Habits?" 2013, accessed February 26, 2015, http://www.apa.org/news/press/releases/stress/2013/highlights.aspx

68. American Psychological Association: "Self-Esteem That's Based on External Sources Has Mental Health Consequences, Study Says," 2002, accessed February 1, 2015, http://www.apa.org/monitor/dec02/selfesteem.aspx.

69. Harvard Women's Health Watch, "The Health Benefits of Strong Relationships," *Harvard Health Publications*, December 1, 2010, accessed March 4, 2015. http://www.health.harvard.edu/newsletter article/the-benefits-of-strong-relationships.

70. Rush University Medical Center, "Higher Levels of Social Activity Decrease the Risk of Cognitive Decline," Science Daily, 2011, accessed March 14, 2015. http://www.sciencedaily.com/releases/2011/04/110425173906.htm.

71. Wikipedia s.v., "Victim Mentality," last modified June 8, 2015, http://en.wikipedia.org/wiki/Victim_mentality.

72. PBS. "What Is Resilience?", accessed February 19, 2015. http://www.pbs.org/thisemotionallife/topic/resilience/what-resilience.

73. Alexandra Sifferlin, "Study Finds Those Who Feel Younger Might Actually Live Longer," *Time* online, 2014, accessed March 30, 2015. http://time.com/3634042/study-finds-those-who-feel-younger-might-actually-live-longer.

74. "Resilience, Recovery, Primary Prevention and Health Promotion," *New Horizons in Health: An Integrative Approach*, 2001, accessed March 7, 2015. http://www.ncbi.nlm.nih.gov/books/NBK43790.

75. Ibid.

76. Brad Waters, "10 Traits of Emotionally Resilient People," *Psychology Today* online, 2012, accessed March 16, 2015, https://www.psychologytoday.com/blog/design-your-path/201305/10-traits-emotionally-resilient-people.

77. Harvard Men's Health Watch, "Walking: Your Steps to Health," Harvard Health Publications, 2009, http://www.health.harvard.edu/newsletter_article/Walking-Your-steps-to-health.

78. Paul Williams and Paul Thompson, "Walking versus Running for Hypertension, Cholesterol and Diabetes Mellitus Risk Reduction," *Arteriosclerosis, Thrombosis, and Vascular Biology*, 33, no. 5 (2013).

79. American Psychological Association, "American Psychological Association Survey Shows Money Stress Weighing on American's Health Nationwide," 2015, http://www.apa.org/news/press/releases/2015/02/money-stress.aspx.

80. American Psychological Association, "Stress in America," 2014. http://www.apa.org/news/press/releases/stress.

81. Ibid.

82. United Health Group, *Doing Good Is Good for You: 2013 Health and Volunteering Study*, http://www.unitedhealthgroup.com/~/

media/UHG/PDF/2013/UNH-Health-Volunteering-Study. ashx.

83. Terri Cole, "Health Benefits of Volunteering," accessed March 18, 2015, http://www.huffingtonpost.com/terricole/volunteer-ing-health_b_2189477.html.

84. Peter Orszag, "Retirement Will Kill You," *Bloomberg View*, 2013, http://www.bloombergview.com/articles/2013-06-11/retirement-will-kill-you.

85. Gabriel Sahlgren, "Work Longer, Live Healthier," Institute of Economic Affairs, 2013, accessed March 19, 2015, http://www.iea.org.uk/sites/default/files/in-the-media/files/Work%20Longer,%20Live_Healthier.pdf.

86. Dhaval Dave, Inas Rashad, and Jasmina Spasojevic. "The Effects of Retirement on Physical and Mental Health Outcomes," National Bureau of Economic Research Working Paper No. 12123, 2008.

87. Shan Tsai, Judy Wendt, Robin Donnelly, Geert de Jong, and Farah Ahmed, "Age at Retirement and Long Term Survival of an Industrial Population: Prospective Cohort Study," *BMJ*, 2005, http://www.bmj.com/content/331/7523/995.

88. http://www.nimh.nih.gov/health/topics/attention-deficit-hyperactivity-disorder-adhd/index.shtml.

89. Visit Wikipedia's list of genetic disorders at http://en.wikipedia.org/wiki/List_of_genetic_disorders.

90. NHS Choices, "How Genetic Conditions Are Inherited," 2014, accessed March 30, 2015, http://www.nhs.uk/Conditions/Genetics/Pages/Facts.aspx.

91. National Institute on Health, "Can We Prevent Aging?" www.nihseniorhealthgov. 2013, accessed March 29, 2015. http://www.nia.nih.gov/health/publication/can-we-prevent-aging.

92. "Life Expectancy, United States," Data360, accessed March 29, 2015. http://www.data360.org/dsg.aspx?Data_Set_Group_Id=195.

93. Mayo Clinic, 2013, accessed February 25, 2015. http://www.mayoclinic.org/healthy-living/healthy-aging/in-depth/dhea/art-20045605?pg=2.

94. Aimee Picchi, "How Many Americans Make It to 100?" CBS Money Watch, 2014, accessed March 30, 2015. http://www.cbsnews.com/news/how-many-americans-make-it-to-100.

CPSIA information can be obtained
at www.ICGtesting.com
Printed in the USA
LVOW10s0807250318

571066LV00031B/770/P